USING RESEARCH IN PRACTICE

Using Research in Practice

It sounds good, but will it work?

Jaqui Hewitt-Taylor

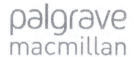

First published 2011 by
PALGRAVE MACMILLAN

Palgrave Macmillan in the UK is an imprint of Macmillan Publishers Limited, registered in England, company number 785998, of Houndmills, Basingstoke, Hampshire RG21 6XS.

Palgrave Macmillan in the US is a division of St Martin's Press LLC, 175 Fifth Avenue, New York, NY 10010.

Palgrave Macmillan is the global academic imprint of the above companies and has companies and representatives throughout the world.

Palgrave® and Macmillan® are registered trademarks in the United States, the United Kingdom, Europe and other countries.

ISBN 978–0–230–27864–6

This book is printed on paper suitable for recycling and made from fully managed and sustained forest sources. Logging, pulping and manufacturing processes are expected to conform to the environmental regulations of the country of origin.

A catalogue record for this book is available from the British Library.

A catalog record for this book is available from the Library of Congress.

To John, age 5, who helped me to decide on the title for this book.

'Mummy, what are you doing?'
'Trying to decide what to call the book I'm writing.'
'Oh ... what's it about?'
'I guess it's about ... how we decide on the best way to try to stop people from being poorly.'
'Has it got any trains in it?'
'Uh ... no. Not really.'
'Well, I'd call that boring then!'

Contents

List of Tables and Figures   xi

Part I   What is research, and why should it be used?

1   **Why should we use research?**   3
    The benefits of using research   3
    The challenges involved in using research   5
    Summary   8

2   **What is research?**   9
    Defining research   9
    Research language   11
    Research, audit and clinical evaluation   11
    Research paradigms   13
    Methodologies and methods   15
    Summary   16

Part II   Is the research any good?

3   **Finding information**   19
    Where to look for information   19
    Deciding what information you need   21
    Identifying key words   22
    Boolean and, or and not   24
    Truncation and Wildcards   25
    Searching in the right field   26
    Recording the results of searches   26
    Summary   27

4   **Appraising research**   29
    Why research needs to be appraised   29
    What the research is about   31
    Literature review   31

Methodology   32
Methods   32
Sampling   33
Ethical considerations   36
Analysis   38
Reliability and validity   38
Results and findings   39
Conclusions and recommendations   39
Is the study is applicable?   40
Using existing frameworks to evaluate research   40
Summary   41

5 **Appraising quantitative research**   **46**
The principles of quantitative enquiry   46
Practice situations in which quantitative enquiry
is likely to be useful   46
Research question/hypothesis   47
Research design/methodology   48
Sampling   51
Methods of data collection   51
Reliability and validity   52
Data analysis   53
Results   59
Conclusions and recommendations   60
Application to practice   60
Summary   61

6 **Appraising qualitative research**   **65**
Principles of qualitative enquiry   65
Situations in which qualitative enquiry may be useful   65
Research question   66
Literature review   66
Methodology   67
Methods   68
Sampling   71
Data analysis   72
Truth of data   73
Findings   76
Conclusions   76
Applying qualitative research to practice   76
Summary   77

7 **Appraising mixed methods research**   **81**
The principles of mixed methods research   81
When mixed methods research may be useful?   83

What is the research about?   83
Literature review   83
Methodology   84
Methods of data collection   85
Sample   86
Ethical issues   86
Data analysis   87
Findings   88
Conclusions and recommendations   89
Quality in mixed methods research   89
Applying mixed methods research to practice   90
Summary   90

8   Using summaries of evidence   94
Using summaries of evidence   94
Systematic reviews   95
Meta analysis   99
Meta synthesis   104
Mixed methods synthesis   107
Clinical guidelines   107
Hierarchies of evidence   109
Summary   110

Part III   Putting research into practice

9   Making decisions   115
What you need to make a decision   115
Patient experiences and preferences   118
Making the 'right' decision   121
Explaining and defending your decisions   122
Summary   122

10 Changing your practice   123
Deciding what you want to change   123
Aims or objectives   125
Planning what you will do   126
Resources   127
Barriers to change   128
Timetable   129
Evaluating your new practice   129
Planning for sustained change   129
Defending your practice   130
Action planning   130
Summary   131

11   Changing team practice   **132**
    Deciding on what needs to be changed   133
    Ways to approach change management   133
    Force field analysis   134
    Barriers to change   135
    Key players   138
    Readiness for change   140
    Changing practice   141
    Motivating managers to allow changed practice   142
    Changing multidisciplinary practice   143
    Summary   145

12   Evaluating new practice   **146**
    What should be evaluated?   146
    When to evaluate?   147
    Approaches to evaluation   148
    Evaluation methods   149
    Who or what to collect information from?   151
    Who should gather data?   151
    Biases   152
    When to collect data?   153
    Interpreting data   153
    Ethics and evaluation   154
    Sharing the findings   155
    Planning ongoing change   155
    Summary   156

Conclusion   157

Appendix 1: Deciding whether to use a study's findings   159

Appendix 2: Was an appropriate statistical test used?   162

Appendix 3: Action plan template examples   163

Appendix 4: Additional resources   164

References   166

Index   179

List of Tables and Figures

Tables

3.1	Examples of search terms which Amelie might use	23
A2.1	Are the data parametric or non-parametric?	162
A3.1	Project aim	163
A3.2	Goal	163

Figures

5.1	Diagram of a bell-shaped curve	54
8.1	Diagrammatic representation of a Forest plot	101

Part I

What is research, and why should it be used?

Why should we use research?

Every year or so, the folk who deal with TV licensing try to persuade me ('the occupier') to buy a TV licence. However, the small library of leaflets that I have acquired from them, detailing my options for procuring a license, accompanied by threats about what fate awaits me if I continue to decline one, does not answer this question: as I do not have a TV, why do I need a TV license, and what benefits would owning one bring me? (Getting a TV is now out of the question, because my correspondence with TV licensing is such fun, and they occasionally call by personally to see how I'm doing with getting my license. I'd miss them if I had a TV, and the license to go with it.)

The moral of the story of my TV non-license is: if you are being asked to do something, you usually want to know why you should do it. So, it makes sense to start by thinking about why it might be a good idea to use research, before getting into the practicalities of doing so.

The benefits of using research

The reasons that are put forward for using research in practice are usually related to it being beneficial for patients (Department of Health, 2008; Gifford *et al.*, 2007). This seems like a good reason, but it begs the question of how healthcare professionals using research is beneficial to patients. Basing care on good evidence should logically improve care and, as Chapter 2 will discuss, information which is generated from research is often considered to be a good source of evidence, so using it should improve care. However, for research to be useful, it has to be of good enough quality to merit use, and relevant to what it is being used for. Using research whose conclusions and recommendations are dangerously wrong will not be beneficial. Equally, if research is applied in the wrong context, it will not necessarily be helpful.

A very good piece of research about assessing pain in children aged four to seven might not be particularly useful to transfer to assessing pain in a two-year old. Saying that using research can improve patient care is true, but only if it is reasonable quality research, and used in the right place, for the right thing.

The benefits which using research brings to patients are often seen in terms of people having access to the best type of treatment or care. However, using research, where appropriate, can also be beneficial to individuals other than the person receiving care. Giving the most effective drug to a person with Chronic Obstructive Pulmonary Disease might improve their quality of life, and also mean that their family enjoys a better quality of life. In addition, they might be admitted to hospital less frequently, and other patients therefore have to wait less time for admission. They might require less additional drugs and General Practitioner consultations, freeing up resources for others. The counterargument to this is that if research shows a very expensive treatment to be the best option, it is distressing for people to whom this is not available because of the cost, or brings benefit to some individuals but reduces the resources available for others. Debates about justice in healthcare provision are a lot more complex than just whether or not research should be used, but using research can sometimes be beneficial for individuals, and society as a whole. It therefore makes sense to at least consider what the research says when making decisions.

Using research has the potential to improve job satisfaction: knowing that we are using what have been found to be the best approaches to care can improve the level of satisfaction we have in our work. Research may also show the most effective way of working, and even when this means taking time to learn to do something in a different way, it may be more efficient in the long term and make our working lives easier.

One of the benefits of using research, or perhaps being seen to use research, may have nothing to do with individual patients or personal job satisfaction, but be linked with a profession as a whole being viewed in a more positive light. If an occupational group can successfully claim that it's work is based on a significant research element, their claim to professionalism may be greater (Webber, 2009). Whether this is a useful claim, and whether it should be a strong driver to use research in everyday practice, is debatable. It might not seem a terribly good reason to go around looking for research to use on a busy shift when the status of the profession is not, at that precise moment, your number one concern. However, it can be a powerful incentive for some members of occupational groups and may be one of the corporate drivers for using research in practice.

The main benefits of using research, then, are the benefits to individuals and, by association, to society as a whole; increased job satisfaction for staff; and a profession which uses research to inform its practice having a better standing. If this is the case, it might seem strange that research is consistently reported to be underused in practice (Björkström and Hamrin, 2001;

Bonner and Sando, 2008; Brenner, 2005; Chau *et al.*, 2008; Gerrish and Clayton, 2004; Hutchinson and Johnston, 2004; Karlsson and Tornquist, 2007; Kuuppelomaki and Tuomi, 2005; Morris-Docker *et al.*, 2004; Scott *et al.*, 2008; Sitzia, 2002; Thompson *et al.*, 2006). However, there are plenty of things that make using research difficult, and many reasons why it is not always the number one priority for practitioners, even when it is on their 'desirable' list.

The challenges involved in using research

Notwithstanding the benefits of using research, getting around to finding research about a practice issue, checking it's quality and making any necessary changes in practice because of it often falls off the end of an ever-expanding 'to do' list. This is partly because of time constraints and more pressing or obvious priorities (Bonner and Sando, 2008; Brenner, 2005; Chau *et al.*, 2008; Gerrish and Clayton, 2004; Hutchinson and Johnston, 2004; Karlsson and Tornquist, 2007; Thompson *et al.*, 2006), because finding information can seem difficult, and the language of research appears complex and confusing (Clifford *et al.*, 2001; Burton 2004; Hutchinson and Johnston, 2004; Hart *et al.*, 2008). One aspect of this book, perhaps the main one, is to make reading research less complex for those who are trying to decide whether or not to use it in practice.

Finding information is often the first challenge in using research. You might have had the experience of doing a search and drawing a complete blank, when you knew that there must be information out there on your chosen subject. Alternatively, you may have done what seemed a perfectly sensible search and got a whole list of things that you really could not see as being anything to do with your request, or may have been presented with so much information that you felt you could never even begin to look at it all. Chapter 3 aims to make searching for information make more sense, and to explain why when you ask for 'children and pain', you can get 4760 articles, most of which seem only very vaguely related to your search, with the 27 on pain in children lost somewhere in the pile.

Once you have gathered information, it can be difficult to know whether to act on what you have read. Sometimes what puts people off using research is the thought of wading through papers which are full of polysyllabic words which once bounced around them in the haze of a post-lunch lecture in a warm classroom. However, most healthcare professionals can and probably do understand research well enough to use it: you just may not know the particular terminology as well as you do other terminology. Research terminology can seem very convoluted and complex, but the ideas behind it are not. One of the intentions of this book is to simplify the language which is used in reporting research. For people who have the time to spend hours pouring over articles, or for whom it is their whole job, the complexities of research may be a delight. This book is aimed at people who probably do not see it that way, or who do not have the time or inclination for that, and who, despite wanting to give the best possible care, do not want to be up until midnight before an early shift trying to understand the sub categories of methodologies. It is aimed at those who want to be able to read research reports, and decide whether or not to use the recommendations from them in practice, but not take a lead role in designing and conducting research studies. To draw a parallel to travel: when I am planning to go somewhere, I like to know where the place I am thinking of going is, what languages are spoken there, whether it is snowy, hot, mountainous, flat, has good beaches or diving options and whether there are any other relevant issues such as civil war that could influence my visit. That is pretty much what I need to know to decide: whether to go or not, how long the flight will be, whether to pack hiking boots, ski jacket, mask and snorkel, beach gear etc. and whether I can get by in my versions of English, Spanish or French. However, I don't especially feel the need to know the plate tectonics of the location, how the climate has come to be that way or the history behind the languages spoken. My husband usually knows all this, so

a. It would be churlish not to use his knowledge.
b. I am not that interested in the detail, because I do not need to know it to make the decisions I have to make.
c. If I happen to decide to move there, I can find the extra details when (and if) I need them.

Similar points can apply to research: you can probably decide whether or not to use a piece of research without having to know all the ins and outs of why and how it came to be that way. You may just need to know what things mean in terms of what you should do about them, and there are a lot of things that you can find out about in more detail on a 'need-to-know basis'. Chapters 4–7 give a basic and simplified overview of what to look for in research studies and how to decide if they are any good or not. But they are at my holiday-planning level, not my husband's.

Perhaps a more difficult decision though is this: if a piece of research seems to be of good quality, should you take the plunge and use it? (Clifford *et al.*, 2001; Sitzia, 2002; Carrion, Woods and Norman, 2004; Hutchinson and Johnston, 2004; Hart *et al.*, 2008) Deciding that a piece of research looks good on paper is one thing, but deciding to use it where you work is another thing altogether. A really good piece of research is also only useful in situations that it is appropriate for, so a challenge in using research effectively is not just deciding whether a study is 'good' or not, but thinking about whether your situation is the right time and place to use it. You might work in a medical ward which mostly deals with long-term respiratory problems and be reading some research about people are who are hospitalized with long-term conditions. If this was carried out with people who have long-term neurological conditions, whether or not it would apply to your work situation depends on exactly what the research was about. If it was a clinical trial about a new drug for Multiple Sclerosis, the chances are that it is not relevant to most of the practice in your unit. However, if it is about the concerns which people with long-term conditions have regarding loss of independence when they are hospitalized, then it may be very relevant, even though the medical conditions which the participants have are completely different.

Once you have decided whether the research is relevant, you still have to put other things into the melting pot of decision making. Using even the highest quality research, in the right context, but in isolation from all other considerations, is rarely a good idea, and Chapters 8 and 9 in particular will discuss the importance of research being a part, but not the entirety, of decision making. If you decide that what you have read is applicable to your area and you really should use it, the hardest part is often yet to come. Doing whatever you have in theory decided to do and perhaps encouraging others to do too is often much more difficult than deciding that it really does seem a good idea. Using established practice may not be the best option, but it often feels much safer than risking the uncertainty which attempting to change practice in order to reflect research findings can create (Scott *et al.*, 2008). There is always a risk that a new approach will not work, and changing practice carries a risk, takes time and often presents challenges. This, along with a lack of time and heavy workloads, can make using research seem insurmountable (Bonner and Sando, 2008; Brenner, 2005; Chau *et al.*, 2008; Gerrish and Clayton, 2004; Hutchinson and Johnston, 2004; Karlsson and Tornquist, 2007; Morris-Docker, 2004; Sitzia, 2002; Thompson *et al.*, 2006). It may also be difficult to know, practically, how to change your own or other people's practice and to have the confidence to do so. For this reason, Chapters 10–11 deal with the practicalities of changing practice in the light of research findings.

Finally, a point which is often missed is evaluating new practice. If the aim of using research is primarily to improve healthcare in some way, then you really need to know if this has been achieved, not just whether something new is being done. Something which sounds as if it should work may not, and something which seems to work may actually not be as good as it seems. Equally, when you are orchestrating a change in practice, it can seem like all hard work and listening to whingeing, but an evaluation may show benefits which makes your suffering seem entirely (or at least very slightly) worthwhile. It can also be useful for colleagues, managers and budget holders to know whether a new approach has had positive outcomes or not, as this may motivate continued participation or resource investment. It is always important to evaluate any new practice, and Chapter 12 deals with this aspect of using research.

Summary

This book is written for those who want to be able to find research that is relevant to their practice, decide with some confidence whether or not to use it and, if the decision is yes, to do so. It may be useful for undergraduate students, some post graduate students (especially those who are looking at evaluating evidence to use in practice, rather than conducting their own research) and for those not doing any academic study but want to read more about using evidence to inform their practice.

The book is divided into three parts: Chapters 1 and 2 deal with the background of why you might want to use research and what it is; Chapters 3–8 deal with making decisions about the quality of research, deciding where and when to use research and incorporating other types of evidence into clinical decisions; and Chapters 9–12 deal with implementing research in practice or changing practice. Chapters 3–8 begin with an example of a practice situation, and use this throughout the rest of the chapter to illustrate some of the points made. At the end of each chapter in this section a worked example or two are given, to consolidate the points made in the chapter.

What is research?

2

When you are looking for something, it is usually fairly helpful to know what it is you are looking for. So, before talking too much about finding and using research, it seems a good idea to clarify what research is.

Defining research

The main themes in definitions of research are that it is a systematic process, in which information is gathered and analysed, resulting in knowledge being generated (Burton, 2004; Le May, 2001). That might be completely new knowledge, knowledge that confirms what was already suspected or known, or knowledge that adds to the picture of what is already known. It might be a huge leap in knowledge, or a tiny piece of a jigsaw of knowledge, but it adds to existing knowledge in some way.

If research is about generating knowledge, then what is it about research that makes it different from, or better than, other ways of finding things out? That may not always be easy to see, because the term research is used in many different ways in everyday life, some of which are not, strictly speaking, accurate ways of using the term. When I am trying to find the best flight for my next vacation, I might say I am 'researching' the options. However, whether I am really researching the options, or just checking them out and finding what seems, on a cursory search, to be the best deal, is debatable. One of the distinctions between research and other ways of gathering information is that research should use a systematic process. This means that the way in which information is sought is carefully thought out, designed to make sure that nothing is missed, and that the way in which that information is analysed creates as much certainty as possible that it is fully and accurately interpreted. The distinction between me searching for flights and really researching them might be: whether I look at the ten or so sites which I usually use to book flights and see which seems to be the best option (checking it out); or use every possible way of getting information on flights to conduct an exhaustive trawl, and then look into the very fine detail of exactly what this information means, so that I am about 99.99 per cent certain that I have the best deal on all counts (closer to research). It is very easy to miss information, or to not get the full picture if you are not systematic, and finding and analysing information systematically is more likely to mean that the results and conclusions drawn from it are right, true or accurate.

What constitutes a systematic approach to gathering information depends on what information is being sought. The best approach to finding out whether a new drug is safe and does what it is intended to do is very different from the best way of finding out how it feels to be the sibling of a child with cerebral palsy. However, in both cases, the difference between doing research and other ways of gathering and analysing information is that the processes followed in research should be systematic and rigorous. This should mean that there is a good level of certainty that nothing was missed, and that the way the information was gathered, and how decisions were made about what the information meant, gives as accurate a representation as possible of the subject in question.

It can be useful to use tried-and-tested ways of doing research, because, in this case, what needs to be considered to make sure that the information is gathered and analysed systematically has already been thought out and agreed. For example, for drugs trials, the tried-and-tested technique of a Randomized Controlled Trial (RCT) (see Chapter 5) is often used. Because the basic structure for this technique exists, when a new drug needs to be tested, the research team involved can slot their study into the tried-and-tested structure, adapting it to fit exactly what they are testing, but knowing the things that they need to consider in their research protocol. This is not to say that new and innovative approaches cannot be used, but often tried-and-tested ways are used because they are known to work.

As well as the process of gathering information needing to be systematic for it to be considered to be 'research', the process has to be the right one for the job. The right approach to gathering information depends on what the research is about. If the intention of a study is to find out whether or not it is advisable to let parents be with their children in the recovery room following surgery, the best approach to this depends on what aspect of the child's well-being is being considered. If the main concern is the child's physical safety and health, it would be useful to use a research design that allows a comparison of the vital signs, incidence of adverse incidents and time to return safely to the ward for matched groups of children who do and do not have their parents with them in the recovery room. However, if the main concern is how parents feel about being with or away from their child, then an approach which focuses on looking in some depth at their subjective experiences of being with or not being with their child would be more appropriate. It might be ideal to consider both, and that might be a form of 'mixed methods' research (see Chapter 7): because two different approaches might need to be used within one study. So, research should use an appropriate, systematic approach to generating knowledge. However, because research gets dressed up in special terminology, it can seem more complex than that.

Research language

It can seem that in order to read research reports you have to learn a whole new language, which is unnecessarily complex. It probably is, but that is no different from any other group of terms, or language. Car mechanics have their own language, which is incomprehensible to people like me. I once had a beautiful Renault 5, which was clunking away more than usual; so I called a garage, where the mechanic told me that it sounded as if the wheel bearings were worn. He did not seem too bothered though, so I drove from Sheffield to Southampton, carrying with me as much of the contents of our house as a Renault 5 can take. The next day, the wheels began to act in a way that was curiously unrelated to the steering wheel, and the error of my understanding of 'worn wheel bearings' became apparent. It might have been more useful if the mechanic had said: 'The things that make your wheels do what the steering wheel says are pretty nearly shot to pieces, and if you do not have them fixed you may go to the intensive care complex where you are scheduled to start work rather faster than you anticipated.' If he had said that, I am pretty sure I would have understood, and might not have decided to use my car as a removal lorry.

Research language is no different from any other language or 'trade speak': it is the language that people have developed to talk about research, and what is actually happening is easily understood, if you can get past the terminology. It is also important to decide what level you want to understand at. Do you want to know the research equivalent of whether having worn wheel bearings matters particularly, or do you want to know how to get hold of new ones and fix the car yourself? If the former, you probably do not have to worry about all the nuances of terminology and technical specifications in as much depth as you do to achieve the latter.

Research, audit and clinical evaluation

A common question is 'what is the difference between research, audit and clinical evaluation?' The reality is that there is not always an absolute and clear cut difference which everyone agrees on (Wade, 2005). The processes being followed by research, audit and clinical evaluation all aim to generate knowledge, and they all gather and analyse relevant types of information (or data) to achieve this. The standards expected are, or should be, as high for all (Wade, 2005). The National Patient Safety Agency and Research Ethics Service (2008) suggest that one distinction between the three is that research aims to create new knowledge, audit to produce information to direct the delivery of high-quality care (which could be seen as new knowledge about how care is being delivered) and service evaluation to define or judge current care (which could be considered to be new knowledge about current care). So, although they all aim to produce different types of knowledge, one could say that they all aim to produce information or knowledge, which is likely, in its own way, to be new.

The difference between the three is perhaps more in the nature of the knowledge being generated than in its novelty. Wade (2005) suggests that research investigates what should be done, whereas audit investigates whether or not what was thought to be done is being done and possibly why this is. Research might show whether or not a new drug is effective for treating acute asthma in children, whereas an audit might show whether staff in Accident and Emergency departments prescribe this drug to children who attend with acute asthma.

One further distinction between research, audit and clinical evaluation may be that some forms of research involve testing new interventions, with a view to using them in the future, whereas audit and clinical evaluation only involve an intervention or interventions which are already in use (National Patient Safety Agency and Research Ethics Service, 2008). In research, the intervention occurs because of the research, whereas in audit or clinical evaluation, the intervention would happen anyway, but some aspect of it is evaluated or audited.

The distinction between research, audit and clinical evaluation is nonetheless not always clear cut. If a new drug for treating angina is being tested, and people who arrive in Accident and Emergency with angina and who consent to be in the study are randomly allocated to a test group that is given the new drug or a control group that is given the usual drug, then that is almost certainly research. A new intervention is being given, for the purpose of seeing if it works, and patients are being put into groups and given the intervention or not because of the research. Some get a drug that they would not otherwise get and others do not get the drug that they would usually get; so something changes in how they are treated. In contrast, if a protocol exists which says that a certain drug should be given to people who present with angina, then a study which evaluates whether this happens or not is probably audit or evaluation because the people with angina get the drug they would get anyway, and the investigation is checking whether they get what is recommended or not. However, if the investigation goes on to ask medical staff why they prescribe what they do, it might be less clear if that is a piece of research, or an extension of the audit activities. It might be considered audit if it was done as part of an audit of what is given and why, but if it was a stand-alone piece of work, purely looking at how physicians make this decision, it might be considered research. So, the answer is not always absolute.

For some purposes, the distinction of research, audit and clinical evaluation is important. However, if you want to use existing evidence to inform your practice, perhaps what matters most is not what the label says the study is, in terms of whether it is research, audit or clinical evaluation, but whether what was done was ethical, what information was being sought and whether this information was appropriately and systematically gathered and analysed.

Research paradigms

The best way to find something depends on what it is you are trying to find. There are as many ways of carrying out research as there are subjects to investigate, and what a researcher aims to find should direct the way in which their study is designed and conducted. If a study aims to find which shop sells the cheapest ice cream, a definite, measurable, numerical answer is required. The approach taken to finding this would need to be one which assumes cost, expressed in numbers, to be all important, and in which, regardless of how the ice cream looks or tastes, only the cost matters. So, the design would have to fit a 'belief' that a numerical measure of cost is the way to 'generate knowledge' about ice cream. It would be of no value, for that particular study, to have people wax lyrical about the texture and taste of various flavours, because, while these may be important (and I believe they are), that is not what the study is all about. That would be useful for another study, about the quality of ice cream.

These 'beliefs' or philosophical assumptions about what type of information is important are the basis of what are referred to as research paradigms. Research paradigms are influenced by beliefs about the nature of reality (ontology), ideas about knowledge (epistemology), the values which underpin the research (axiology) and the nature of the processes used to gain knowledge (methodology) (MacInnes, 2009). There are, usually described as being, two main research paradigms: quantitative and qualitative (see Chapters 5 and 6).

Quantitative research, sometimes also referred to as positivist research, quantifies things, so it uses numbers. It also sees truth as objective, not dependent on context or interpretation (Lee, 2006a; McGrath and Johnson, 2003; Sale, Lohnfeld and Brazil, 2002; Tarling and Crofts, 2000). In quantitative research, the paradigm, or belief underpinning the research, is that, by using numbers, one can show whether something works or not, and can predict how likely it is that this should apply, equally, to most people within a certain population or group (referred to as generalizability) (Lee, 2006a). A paradigm for investigating which shop sells the cheapest ice cream would be quantitative: one which takes the stance that knowledge about ice cream can be developed in a measurable and numerical way, which sees it as possible and desirable to produce a result which can be applied across a whole population, and which sees the cost of ice cream as important. If I carried out a good quantitative study to identify which place sells the cheapest ice cream, I should be able to send everyone I know there with a high degree of certainty that they would all be charged the same price and get the cheapest possible ice cream. This approach is important when it is necessary to know that a specific action is likely to be safe, or the best option, for almost everyone within a population. For example, to check that a new drug is likely to have the desired effect, and minimal side effects, for most people, or that a way of scanning is likely to detect any important changes in the vast majority of cases.

Qualitative research, which is also sometimes referred to as 'naturalistic' or 'interpretivist' research engages with words rather than numbers, and does not aim to quantify things (Kearney, 2005; Goodman, 2008). It looks at the meaning of human experiences and acknowledges that 'truth' may be subjective and interpreted differently by different people or in different circumstances (Lo Bindo-Wood and Haber, 2005). Qualitative research does not aim to find an answer which can be confidently applied to everyone in a given population (so qualitative studies do not usually aim to achieve generalizability). Instead, the researcher builds up a picture of what is being studied, and the context of the study, so that those reading the description can decide how far this might apply to their situation, or the population they are thinking of applying it to. This paradigm is often used to enhance understanding of individual and subjective things like feelings, values or beliefs. If I wanted to find out which shop sells the best ice cream (and I believe I have), the qualitative paradigm would probably be the most appropriate. It would be unreasonable for me to expect that I could direct everyone to my best ice cream with confidence that they would agree with me. Unless you like *dulce de leche*, you would not like my best tasting ice cream. Also, this particular shop only sells it in waffle cones; so if waffle cones are not to your liking, then it would not work for you. If you like polite portions, then this is definitely not for you. However, if you like big dollops of *dulce de leche* ice cream, creamy, full fat and with little drizzles of *dulce de leche* in it, in a choco-late coated waffle cone, then I would suggest you go to the store halfway along the road behind the bus station in Puerto Iguazú in Argentina, and indulge. Even then, you might be disappointed, because what exactly makes ice cream yummy is hard to determine. You would also need to hear the context of my study because on an icy January day in England, it might not seem as delicious as it did on a sunny day in South America, when I had spent the day wander-ing around the Iguazú falls, and was planning an evening lying in my hammock watching the stars.

There is also an increasing interest in what are referred to as 'mixed methods' of research or 'mixed methodologies' (Bryman, 2006; Halcomb, Andrew, Brannen, 2009). This is often described as a third paradigm, or the 'pragmatic' paradigm (see Chapter 7), but it basically means that a study uses a combination of qualitative and quantitative approaches in some way.

In practice, a good quality piece of quantitative research about the best way to secure arterial lines in children might be applicable to most children on a paediatric intensive care unit (PICU). However, a piece of research about par-ents' experiences of their child requiring intensive care admission would not be something that could be so easily applied to all parents whose child was on PICU. You cannot so easily and precisely hand out what might be described as psychosocial and emotional support to everyone as you can arterial line dress-ings. In addition, people's emotions and circumstances and their responses to these are not so easy to know as the state of an arterial line. The research about parents' experiences will give useful pointers and considerations, but this is more complex to apply and requires a lot more consideration of the context and indi-vidual involved than whether or not an arterial line is suitable for a 'standard' dressing.

Qualitative and quantitative research are equally valuable, but it is important that each is used appropriately. In terms of ice cream, I would definitely be of the opinion that the qualitative aspects of knowledge are the most important. However, if my son ever needs medical intervention, I will want to know that whatever treatment is proposed is pretty much proven to be the best option before proceeding. So, in that situation, I would want high-quality quantitative evidence. Both paradigms are important, and have a place, they just need to be used for the right thing.

Methodologies and methods

Research paradigms are related to the set of beliefs or values which underpin the research, but no two subjects are exactly the same, so within each paradigm there is a range of possibilities of approaching getting information (Dixon-Woods *et al.*, 2004; Polkinghorne, 2005). These are often referred to as methodologies. So, even if two studies fall within the same paradigm, they may very legitimately use different methodologies. The paradigm is perhaps the way of viewing things, the beliefs or values which underpin the research, and the methodology is the way in which the researcher approaches getting the information (MacInnes, 2009).

If one were to study the quality of ice cream using a qualitative paradigm, the study would be based on the view that knowledge about ice cream cannot be developed numerically and in a way that can be generalized to every ice cream eater in the world. It would accept that ice cream quality concerns abstract and immeasurable issues such as texture, taste, creaminess, personal preference and context of consumption, which not everyone may agree with. The methodology selected could be ethnography, where the researcher immerses himself/herself in a culture of ice cream eating for a considerable period of time (yes please) or phenomenology, where they seek to achieve an in-depth exploration of people's experiences of the phenomenon of ice cream eating (not so attractive to me because I want to get into eating the ice cream myself rather than hearing about it). Ethnography and phenomenology are both qualitative methodologies, but the processes they follow are different (see Chapter 6).

Methodology and paradigm are therefore slightly different things, but they are very closely linked because to get information which fits the paradigm being used, you have to use a methodology that matches that paradigm. Because they are so closely linked, sometimes the words methodology and paradigm are used interchangeably. This may not really matter a great deal for the purpose of reading research reports. It is worth debating in some arenas, but possibly not worth getting too exercised over if you are deciding on the quality of a piece of research, not the semantics of the report. Looking for the term 'methodology', or 'paradigm', or both, and seeing if they fit what is being studied is probably the most important thing.

Having decided on what paradigm and methodology are best, the researcher has to decide on the methods he/she will use: how they will actually get the information they need. If a researcher has decided to find out what parents whose children have eczema think of the information they get about their child's condition, they might decide that this would fall within the qualitative paradigm, use phenomenology as their approach to the research process (methodology), and maybe interviews with parents as the way of collecting information (method). Equally, they might use observation at an eczema clinic to see what information is given and how, and then interview the parents to see what they made of this. So, the methods would then be interviews and observation.

There are some methods which lend themselves to certain paradigms or methodologies. In-depth interviews are linked to the qualitative paradigm and methodologies (see Chapter 6), but some methods can be used in any paradigm or methodology, depending on exactly how they are used. The methods are the tools that you use to gather information or data, and like a lot of tools, they come in different shapes, styles and sizes and can be used for different things. A qualitative study might use in-depth interviews with ten parents. However, in quantitative methodology it might be appropriate to use very short, tick box (yes/no/don't know) interviews with 2000 parents in order to detect trends. The important thing is that the right tool is chosen to get the information that is required, and that it is then used correctly.

Summary

This chapter has described what research is (a systematic and rigorous process of enquiry), and some of the language that goes with it. The paradigm, methodology and methods of gathering and analysing data should be appropriate for the subject being investigated and a good study design is one that uses the right approach to get the type of information it needs.

The next stage is to get information on the subject you are interested in: Chapter 3 deals with searching for information: I am off to Puerto Iguazú for that ice cream meanwhile!

Part II
Is the research any good?

Finding information

3

Scenario

Amelie works in a children's surgical ward. A few weeks ago, she noticed that not many people seem to use the existing pain assessment tool (which consists of a linear scale graded 1–10 for older children, and a smiley face scale graded 1–5 for younger children). There had also been a number of complaints from parents about how their child's pain was managed. Amelie felt that practice related to pain management could be improved, but was unsure where to start. When she asked her colleagues about this, many of them were of the opinion that the existing pain assessment tool was not very useful. Amelie agreed to look into the alternatives. Her first challenge was where and how to look for information.

Where to look for information

The best place to look for information depends on what information you want. Amelie wants information about pain assessment in children, and probably wants this to include relevant research reports on it as well. A database which deals with medical and nursing information, and includes journals which publish research in these fields, would therefore probably be a good place for her to start.

Databases are file structures which are organized in a logical way so that they can be searched, information can be retrieved and they can be managed and updated (Hebda and Czar, 2009). Usually they are named or described in a way that indicates what type of information they contain, so that you can decide whether it is the right database for your subject. Amelie might usefully search the CINAHL (Cumulative Index to Nursing and Allied Health Literature) database because a database devoted to nursing and allied health literature seems likely to contain things related to pain assessment and management. Other databases which she might find useful include PubMed, Medline and EMBASE. Many databases require a subscription to access them fully, and healthcare organizations and universities often have such subscriptions. It would be useful for Amelie to check which databases her organization subscribes to, and whether she has to activate a subscription, because this might affect where she can search and also whether she can retrieve abstracts and full texts of articles from these databases.

There are some electronic frameworks or portals which allow you to search more than one database or resource at a time. For instance, Athens (www.athens. ac.uk) allows you to access a range of databases and electronic resources through one sign-in process: you still need to access the resources separately once you get in, but if you are using resources that are 'on Athens' (or can be accessed through Athens), you only have to sign into the system once. To draw an analogy with real life: if you want to do a whole lot of exercise on machines, have a coffee and then go swimming, you could go to the gym, then go to a coffee shop, then go to the swimming pool. Or you could go to a leisure complex that has a gym, a coffee bar and a swimming pool, and use them all under one roof. Using Athens is like the latter: it means that you can go through one electronic door, and then wander round all the sections that you want to use. You still have to go to different places within Athens for each one, but it is sometimes easier to do it all under one roof. Again, it would be worthwhile for Amelie to check whether her organization subscribes to this type of resource.

Search engines can also be useful, but they are slightly different from databases. When we were looking for flights to Finland last year, I informed my family that I would see what I could find. My son, then aged four, sat in an unusually attentive manner while I typed. After a while, when all I had retrieved were lists of prices, times, dates and other tedious looking things, he asked when the engine would appear. I must have used the term 'search engine' and, as usual, not explained things properly. However, a search engine is like a train, because it chugs through many places on the World Wide Web, searches for what you have asked for and then, if it finds it, brings it back to you. In more technical terms, it is a coordinated set of computer programs which includes a spider (also sometimes called a 'traveller' or 'bot') that goes to every page on every website that it has been given permission to search. It reads it, creates an index or catalogue from the information on those pages, compares this with your search request and sends you a list of, and usually a link to, the page or pages that have the information you asked for (Saba and McCormack, 2001; SOA.com, 2001). Some search engines scan a large portion of the Web. Specialized search engines are selective about which part of the Web they look at, and individual websites often use a search engine that just looks at the content of their own site. This can be a useful way of finding information, but it depends on which search engine you use and its search scope. If you use one that covers the whole Web, you might get the same article 17 times if 17 web pages have listed it. Search engines also only collect things that they find on web pages, so you would not necessarily get a list of articles that is as comprehensive as you would in a database of journal articles. On the other hand, you may get things which have not been included in databases, such as recent conference proceedings, forthcoming conference presentations or unpublished research.

It is a case of deciding what you want to search and thinking about the best place to search for it: sometimes it is a good idea to use a combination of databases, search engines and other very specific locations. Amelie might use Athens to look at CINAHL and other databases, but also do a Google search to see what pain tools other wards or hospitals have decided to share on their websites, and to find recent conference presentations which are not yet in the published literature but which might be useful. If she knows that someone has written a thesis on pain assessment tools for children and wants it, rather than any papers that have been published form it, or wants to check if anyone has written such a thesis, she could go to the index of theses (www.theses.com) to search. It might also be useful for her to search for reviews which have looked at all the evidence on pain assessment in children. Systematic reviews and guidelines are discussed in Chapter 8, but to make sure she had the evidence from these sources Amelie could search in the list of Cochrane Collaboration's systematic reviews (www. cochrane.co.uk/en/index.html) and the list of guidelines and reviews published by organizations such as the National Institute of health and clinical excellence (NICE) (www.nice.org.uk) and the Joanna Briggs Institute for Nursing Reviews (www.joannabriggs.edu.au/about/home.php).

Deciding what information you need

When you want to find information, regardless of where you plan to search, taking some time to think about exactly what you want to search will probably save you time in the long run. It is a bit like going shopping: taking time to decide exactly what you want to buy can seem pointless if you think that you know what you want to buy. Finding a piece of paper and pen to make a list can seem like faff, but if you do not have a list (or a good enough memory), you may come home with a whole load of interesting and even useful items, but not what you need for tea tonight. Then you may have to go back, or try and make whatever you have bought into something that resembles a meal. Similarly, once you have an idea about what you want or need to get information about, the temptation is to go online and get articles at once, especially given the time constraints you are almost certain to have. However, that may well result in you wasting time later on sifting through irrelevant information. You may find what you want, but it might become lost in the heap of irrelevant information that you have collected, and you may lose the will to sort through it all. Apart from the time and effort you would spend weeding out irrelevant things, if you get an interesting-looking but unrelated article, the chances are you will read it. If you have limited time and a project to do, this will use up precious time: much better not to have irrelevant information to start with. There is also the risk of not finding what was required, and you will spend the day searching and reading, but have nothing to show for it. Amelie wants information on pain assessment tools, not information on parents' views on pain management, or the physiology of pain. These might be useful at some stage, but they are not what she needs right now; so her search needs to be focused on pain assessment tools for children.

Equally though, you need the full range of information on a subject before you make a decision. To use the shopping analogy again, you may see something that looks really good and buy it, only to find later that four or five better things were available and you are now stuck with the worst and most expensive option. If you find one useful-looking piece of research and adopt it, you may have missed five or six much more impressive papers which tell you to do exactly the opposite, or recommend a slightly better way of doing things. You may look silly when someone else unearths them, and you might be encouraging suboptimal care based on one paper which is overridden by several others. So, deciding exactly what you want, and then searching diligently for it until you know you have probably unearthed all, or at least most, of the information on that subject is important.

Identifying key words

Having decided exactly what you want to look for, the next thing to do is to state this in words that you can enter into a search facility (such as a database or search engine). It can be useful to start this process by writing a sentence or phrase stating your requirements, to make sure that you really are clear about exactly what it is that you want and that you do not have too big a task (Holland, 2007). Amelie might write:

I want to find research about pain assessment tools that are used for children

That looks quite focused and manageable. If she had said:

I want to find research articles on pain physiology, assessment, and management in children and young people and why healthcare professionals manage pain the way they do,

that looks too big. She would have at least four subjects to look at (the physiology of pain, pain assessment, pain management options and professional attitudes to and beliefs about pain and its management), and possibly at least as two subdivisions of age group (children and young people).

The next step is to identify from that sentence the key words or concepts that you want to search for (Holland, 2007; Thames Valley Literature Review Standards Group, 2006). Using key words or concepts is how search facilities work: they look for the words you ask for in article titles and abstracts (if those are the parts of the articles that you have asked them to look in) and give you a list of the articles whose title or abstracts contain these words. So, although you may have a sentence which describes exactly what you want to look for, you need to reduce it to key words or concepts before entering it into a search facility. If you enter the whole sentence, you may get everything that has any of the words in that sentence. If Amelie typed 'pain assessment tools that are used for children' into some search facility, she would run the risk of getting all the articles whose title or abstract had any of those words in it. Imagine getting every article which contained the words 'that' or 'are' in its abstract. That would be an awful lot.

So, although Amelie might write:

I want to find research about pain assessment tools that are used for children,

her keywords or concepts would perhaps be 'pain', 'assessment tools' and 'children', and those are the terms she would enter into the search facility of the database.

Although you do not want to get lots of irrelevant information, you do want to get all the information that you can on the subject you are looking at. Amelie may have decided to look for 'pain', 'assessment tools' and 'children', but to find all the relevant literature, she also needs to think about what other words people might use for these terms, or how they might be described in journal articles. So, she should think about what other ways there are of stating each keyword. This might include synonyms for the words, or words that are close enough to be considered synonyms for the purpose of the search (Holland 2007; Thames Valley Literature Review Standards Group, 2006). For instance, 'children' might also be covered by the terms 'paediatric', or 'child'. It is also useful to consider what terms and spellings are used in different types of English, such as 'pediatric' and 'paediatric'. Identifying words which are used for the same thing but in different countries, such as Emergency Room and Accident and Emergency, is also advisable, as is identifying acronyms such as ET Tube or ETT for endotracheal tube and using brand and generic drug names, for example, salbutamol and ventolin (Holland, 2007; Thames Valley Literature Review Standards Group, 2006).

Table 3.1 shows how Amelie might list the alternative terms that could be used for the words she identified for her search. Making a list or table for each word can make it easier for you to be sure that you have thought of all the alternatives, and to check that you look for them all.

Having identified these terms, the next step is to use them in a way to get not only all the information you need, but also avoid lots of unrelated articles. If all these terms were put into a search facility in one go without any precautionary

Table 3.1   Examples of search terms which Amelie might use

Keyword 1	Keyword 2	Keyword 3
Pain	Assessment	Children
Discomfort	Evaluation	Paediatric
Hurt	Measurement	Child

action, they would produce an awful lot of articles, many of which would be irrelevant.

Boolean and, or and not

There are three words which can make your search life easier, and save you a lot of time (providing the database that you use supports them). They are referred to as Boolean terms or Boolean *and, or* and *not*. The term Boolean comes from the name of the inventor of this system, George Boole. The logic which he used to create these search options enables you to instruct your search tool about which words you are interested in when they are linked with each other, and to identify any words that you never want to see in your search results (Holland, 2007).

And

Identifying the terms that you want to find means you can search for articles containing these terms, but you seldom want to look at all the articles which contain any of those terms. Amelie wants to look at the concepts of pain, assessment and children, but she would not want all the articles with a mention of pain, assessment or children in the title or abstract, because that would give her all the papers with anything about children in them, all the papers with anything about pain and all the articles which mention assessment of any kind. If she is using a database that supports the use of Boolean terms, she can use the term *and* so that she is only given results that include all of her stated concepts: pain *and* assessment *and* children. That way she will get a paper titled 'Pain assessment in children undergoing surgery' but not 'Pain management following mastectomy', 'Assessment of teenagers admitted with acute asthmatic attacks' or 'Supporting the siblings of children who have long-term health needs'.

Or

The Boolean term *or* allows you to ask the search facility to look for all the words that you have decided mean the same thing, in one go. If Amelie decides that 'pain' means the same as 'discomfort' then she can use the Boolean *or* to search for 'pain *or* discomfort' rather than doing two searches, one for pain and one for discomfort. If she does this, the search tool will locate all the records that contain the word 'pain' and all the records that contain the word 'discomfort' and then combine both groups of records into a single set. So, although the search tool does two searches, Amelie will only have to set up one search and will be presented with one list of all the articles that contain either of those two keywords.

Not

The Boolean term *not* will exclude articles whose titles or abstracts contain words that you do not want to read about (Holland, 2007). If Amelie wants to search for pain assessment in children but does not want to read anything about teenagers, she could ask for pain *and* assessment *and* children *not* adolescents. One thing to be cautious about though is that this option excludes words in preference to including them. So, this search would exclude an article titled 'Pain assessment in children and adolescents' because the *not* outweighs the other words, even though at least one part of that article might be useful for Amelie.

Combining and, or and not in a single search

You can use more than one Boolean term in the same search (Holland, 2007). Getting this right should reduce the chances of either getting masses of irrelevant information or missing lots of important information, and means that you need to search once, not several times. If Amelie searches for pain *or* discomfort *and* assessment, the search tool will first create a set of articles that contains the terms pain and assessment in the title or abstract. It will then add the set of articles containing the words discomfort and assessment. This means that Amelie will be presented with a set of articles that contains either the word 'pain' or 'discomfort' but also contains the word 'assessment'. It saves having to search first for 'pain' and 'assessment' then for 'discomfort' and 'assessment'.

Many databases and some search engines allow you to use Boolean terms, but if you try to use them in a database or search engine that does not support them, you may not get what you want. If you type child *or* children into a search engine that does not support Boolean logic, then you risk getting every website with the word 'or' in it as well as every one with 'child' or 'children'. You also need to check how the search facility wants the Boolean terms presented: they may need to be inserted in capitals, in italics or with inverted commas or something else. Some databases and search engines use their own system to achieve the same as Boolean terms do. So, it is useful to check that your search engine or database supports the use of Boolean terms or uses an equivalent, if slightly modified, system. This often comes up in the 'advanced search' option.

Truncation and Wildcards

Although Amelie wants to search for articles which use the term 'assessment', this term might be presented in different forms in an article title or abstract: pain assessment, assessing pain and how to assess pain. When you search a database, only the words you type in are found, and for Amelie, typing and searching in turn for

Assessment
Assessing
Assessed
Assess

or even typing *or* for every permutation of every word, would be a bit long winded. Fortunately, because all these words share a common stem 'asses', she can, using a process called truncation, use the shortest version of the word with a truncation character (usually a*) to represent a range of endings (Holland, 2007). Entering 'assess*' instructs the search tool to retrieve all the words that begin with 'assess', such as assess, assessment, assessing and assessed.

With other words, one letter within the word may change from time to time: for instance, 'paediatric' becomes 'pediatric' in the move from British to American spelling. Because the word is not truncated, you cannot use the truncation process, but you can instead use a wildcard character, again usually a*, within the word to instruct the search tool to look for any (or no) letter in that space (Holland, 2007), for example, 'paediatric' becomes 'p*ediatric' with a wildcard search to capture both the American and British spellings.

Searching in the right field

When you search for information on a database, you generally get the choice of where you want to look for the words you have requested (which field you want to search in). This usually includes the option of searching for or within the author name, journal name, title or abstract of the article, or the whole article. It is important to get the right one. If Amelie searches for 'children' or 'paediatric' or 'child' in the journal title field, she will retrieve the entire collection of articles from journals containing any of those words in their title, which is a lot. If you are doing a keyword search, you will usually be looking at searching for a keyword in article abstracts and titles, but occasionally you might want to look in the whole article. Also, you can do a search for the name of an author whose work you want to read or for a journal title if you want to find a particular journal. You just need to search in the right place for what you want.

Recording the results of searches

Usually, people helpfully ask if you have a back up of your work after it is irretrievably lost. They then wonder why, instead of thanks for their insightful comment, they get a narrow-eyed stare and no further Christmas cards. This is the kind of thing that we all know about, and which everyone always tells you when it is too late, so you may want to stop reading now, but it is the kind of thing I feel obliged to say. Always keep a record of the things you find and plan to use, and do it in a manner that best suits the way you work and which guards against computer meltdown, or memory card loss. The editor of this book would probably write the word 'hypocrite' on the manuscript, and add something to the effect of how many references I missed out and seemed incapable of locating. I am not suggesting that I do this myself. It is just something that I know is a good idea.

Summary

In summary then, searching diligently for information takes some effort but it is usually effort well spent because it should save you time later on. It is advisable to be clear about what you want to search for, and using the right terms and combination of terms should make your searching life more bearable. You will probably still get some irrelevant articles, but doing this should reduce the chances of getting overwhelmed with information that you do not need and increase the chances of you getting the vast majority of information on your subject without too much difficulty. Once you have retrieved the information you want, it is time to read it and decide whether it is good enough for you to want to act on it. That is where the next chapter starts.

Worked example

Pritpal works on a medical High Dependency Unit (HDU). The unit has been experiencing some problems in arranging the transfer of patients to the wards. There seems to be inconsistency in how the decision to transfer is made, by whom this is agreed and the processes which need to be followed. After discussion within the medical directorate, Pritpal has been given the task of developing a protocol for the transfer of patients from HDU to the ward. One part of her task is to search for information on the subject. How might she go about this?

Ideas

What Pritpal might search for

- Existing guidelines or protocols regarding the transfer of patients from HDU to wards.
- Research about transfer of patients from HDU to wards
- Evaluations of practice on transfer of patients from HDU to wards
- A range of other literature, such as expert opinion, case studies, or reports on transfer of patients from HDU to wards.

Where Pritpal might search

Databases dealing with healthcare such as CINHAL, Ingenta, Medline and OVID, which she might access through a resource such as Athens.

- Databases of guidelines, such as NICE
- A general search engine, such as Google, to locate unpublished local protocols/ guidelines/ recent findings/ conference proceedings, and reports in Trust documents.

Keywords or phrases

Pritpal might develop the statement:
'I want to find information about transferring patients from HDU to the ward.'

Her key words might be:

- Transfer
- HDU
- Ward

The alternative terms which Pritpal might consider using include

- Transfer: movement
- HDU: High Dependency (it may be better for her to use High Dependency rather than High Dependency Unit because article titles might talk about 'transfer from high dependency' rather than including the word 'unit').

However, she does not want all the articles that have 'ward' or 'HDU' or 'transfer' etc. in the title or abstract, and she probably wants to search as efficiently as possible, so she should consider Boolean terms

Boolean terms

Pritpal might want to use Boolean *and*, for example, to create a search for:

- HDU *and* ward *and* transfer so as to only get results which include all three terms.
- She might also use Boolean *or* to include her synonyms in one search: High Dependency *or* HDU *and* transfer
- Pritpal may want to focus on medical high HDUs, so she may consider using Boolean *not* to exclude, surgical HDUs ('HDU *not* surgical') or psychiatric HDUs ('HDU *not* psychiatric').
- She may also want to consider using a truncation: 'transfer*' in order to capture articles whose titles or abstracts include transfer, transferring, and transferred.

Fields to search

It is likely that Pritpal will initially search in the subject field, unless she is looking for the work of a particular writer.

She might also want to limit her search to the last ten years to be sure of getting up to date information.

Appraising research

4

Scenario

Konrad is a Band 6 nurse who works on a 20-bed general ICU which shares facilities with a 14-bed cardiac ICU. He is interested in trying to reduce the level of noise on the unit because he believes that it may be detrimental to patients. Some of the staff on the unit agree that the noise levels may be problematic, many seem quite indifferent and a small number do not agree with him. He has carried out four searches: one on whether noise is an issue in ICUs, one on the causes of noise in ICUs, one on the effects of noise on patients in ICU and one on the ways in which noise can be reduced in the ICU. Now he wants to appraise all the information that he has gathered to see what direction, if any, he should take in attempting to change practice on his unit.

Why research needs to be appraised

Not all information is good, not everything which might look like research actually fulfils the quality standards of research and not all published research is good quality research. We have all probably, at one time or another, been presented with information which was flawed, even if it seemed to be from a reputable source, or which was in essence accurate, but actually quite misleading. My husband's birthday treat in Peru was one such experience.

We had decided to take the bus from Cuzco to Arequipa, an eight-hour journey across austere but beautiful landscape. Having visited most of the tourist offices on the main square to enquire about our options, we selected what seemed to be the best offer. The man in charge of the office issued us with tickets for the next morning (my husband's birthday), showed us a photograph of 'the kind of bus you will be in' and outlined the many benefits of his outfit. These included 'toilets are available on the journey', and 'a nice café' with 'beautiful views' where we would stop for lunch. My husband remarked on what a pleasant birthday he would have. When we arrived at the bus station at seven o'clock the next morning, there were a number of buses which looked just like the one we had been shown; and a little, eld-erly, battered one was at the end of the row. You already know which one was ours.

The information which our friend in the Cuzco travel office gave us was in some respects true: our bus was 'like' the bus he showed us: it had wheels, a driver and seats. At random intervals it made a toilet stop (women uproad, men downroad). We stopped for lunch at a kiosk which offered the choice of stew of uncertain but globular content, plain biscuits or mints. Or, if it was your birthday and you were after a three-course meal, all three. The view was beautiful, and you could certainly enjoy it while standing outside the kiosk eating your lunch if you had thick enough clothing to dine *al fresco*, rather than snuggling back into the bus amidst your new-found close associates. However, we couldn't help feeling we had been slightly misled.

One of our problems was that what we were acting on was not good quality, systematic, research: we had just called into every office on the square and casually questioned the staff about buses to Arequipa. We had also not thought through exactly what the information that we were given meant, whether everyone would be taking it to mean the same thing, and whether the information was intended to be generalized to every bus trip to Arequipa. Konrad will not want the research equivalent of our bus to Arequipa experience. He will want to be fairly certain that any information which he has about noise on ICUs is a true and accurate representation of reality before he invests considerable time and energy in asking his colleagues to change their practice. By checking exactly what the information presented means, whether it seems to be good quality information, and how far it is likely to apply to his work situation, he should be more confident about whether or not the suggestions stand a reasonable chance of working. We failed to do almost all these things on our Arequipa trip, and thus have only ourselves to blame for any inconvenience caused. Both Cuzco and Arequipa are, by the way, beautiful cities, and the journey is spectacular. I would just advise you to take sandwiches.

By the fact that a piece of research has been published you might think that it should be of a reasonable standard, but this may not be the case. The quality of published research varies, and even articles taken from high-quality journals need to be checked before you decide to implement their recommendations (Coughlan, Cronin and Ryan, 2007). There are plenty of published studies which are perfectly good for what they say they are, but which were never intended to be uncritically used by everyone. If Konrad finds a very good study looking at measures to reduce noise in ICUs that was carried out on an eight-bed general ICU, it may only be partially applicable to his unit, because of the differences between the units. Other studies may be intended as small-scale or pilot studies whose aim is to primarily test processes or to develop ideas for further study. So, all published research should be appraised to check what it was supposed to be used for, and its overall quality, before using it.

Appraising information, especially research, often seems quite difficult, but it need not be. This chapter gives an overview of what you should consider when you evaluate any research with a view to using it in practice. Chapters 5 and 6 deal with the specifics of qualitative and quantitative research and Chapter 7 discusses mixed methods research.

What the research is about

It is useful to know fairly early on if the paper you are spending your valuable time reading is actually relevant to your current project, so, one of the first things to check is what the research says it is about (Lee, 2006c). Konrad may think that he has a useful article because the search found him an abstract that includes the terms ICU and noise. However, the paper may actually be about the effects of artificial lighting on ICU patients. The abstract might say that noise, use of day and night artificial lighting and sleep disturbance can all be detrimental to people in ICU, but that the paper is about the effects of almost constant lighting. That makes it irrelevant to Konrad's purposes, even if it is a good piece of research.

The title will give you a good idea of what the research is about, but the detail of this should be stated fairly early on in the paper itself. How the research report states what it is about depends on what type of research it is (Coughlan, Cronin and Ryan, 2007). It might have a hypothesis or question or problem statement or statement of intent. Hypotheses (proposed explanations that are going to be tested in the research) may be used in quantitative enquiry. However, many perfectly good pieces of quantitative research do not have hypotheses because they do not need them (see Chapter 5). In qualitative enquiry hypotheses are not usually used and a statement explaining what the study explores is more usual (see Chapter 6): for example, 'Exploration of ICU staff's views on noise'. What is important is to check what the research says it is about, so that you can decide whether or not to read it and, as you read it, to see if what is presented matches what the study said it was about.

Literature review

It is useful to check what the person doing the research had read about, and how this influenced their study. If Konrad finds a number of papers showing that noise levels on ICUs tend to be unacceptably high, but the literature presented in a study about the effects of noise on ICU patients suggests that noise levels are not problematic, then he might wonder if the researcher was biased towards showing that noise does not really matter. If his own search retrieved 50 articles about noise in ICU, a study whose literature review stated that no information existed on the subject would perhaps make him wonder whether the researcher was very diligent in their preparation, and therefore if the rest of the study was conducted rigorously.

A bonus of checking the background literature in the papers you use is that it might point you to some articles or conference papers that even the best search would miss. It does not replace a diligent search, but it can be reassuring to look at someone else's literature review, and realize that you have all the main articles, and usefully pick up one or two extras.

Methodology

As Chapter 2 described, the paradigm and/or methodology which a research report says was used tells you about the beliefs which underpinned the study, and what the researchers took to be the best way of addressing the issues in question (MacInnes, 2009). The paradigm or methodology used should 'match' the subject being explored and research question: whether or not this is the case influences whether the research is likely to meet its stated aim (Astin, 2009). Konrad might be alerted to a problem if a study states that it has the hypothesis that increased noise levels are associated with raised heart rates in ICU patients, but also describes itself as falling within the qualitative paradigm, or using a qualitative methodology. Qualitative research does not usually involve testing hypotheses; it usually aims to present an in-depth exploration of a matter, accepting subjectivity and not seeking to generalize findings (Goodman, 2008; Kearney, 2005; Lo Bindo-Wood and Haber, 2005), so these two appear incongruent. The paradigm and methodology should also match the approach taken in the rest of the study: if the research claims to fall within the quantitative paradigm or uses quantitative methodology, then the research question, methods, analysis, results and recommendations should match that. If it says that it falls within the qualitative paradigm or uses qualitative methodology, the question, methods, analysis and the way results are presented should match that.

Being clear about the methodology also helps you to know how the results should be used. For example, whether they should be taken to mean that a certain intervention will work in almost every instance of a given situation, as may be the case in quantitative work, or to give in-depth insights which may be transferrable to some other situations depending on the context, as would be the case with qualitative approaches.

If you cannot find the bit that tells you what the paradigm or methodology is fairly early on in a paper, then you may find it later, but if the person presenting the study was not clear on their methodology, then the chances are you will not be, and you will end up not knowing whether the results or conclusions are something you should use or not.

Methods

The paradigm and methodology tell you what type of information the study was looking for, and the overall approach used. The methods tell you the practicalities of how that information was gathered (Astin, 2009). Unless the right methods are used, it is unlikely that the right information will be found. Konrad may find an article describing a quantitative study that measured noise levels on two ICUs over a 24-hour period and compare these. If the methods used were measuring sound and capturing videos of what was going on at the time so that the noise levels could be matched against events, that seems a reasonable way to measure and account for noise; so the methods seem likely to have produced the type of information that the researcher wanted.

The methods used in a study should also fit the methodology. If a study states that it uses qualitative methodology, but the methods are a set of yes/no answers, which are statistically analysed, then those two do not match. There are some methods which are associated with certain methodologies but many methods can fit different methodologies depending on how they are used. Observation could be used in a quantitative study of noise in ICU to match the recorded sound level against events, with no further detail added. However, it could also be used in a qualitative study to observe staff practice, to note the subtleties of what they do and combine this with interviews to find out what they think about noise, how this matches their practice and what impacts on the level of noise, despite people's intentions.

There is often no one single 'right' method for a study, or a method which will be perfect. Face-to-face interviews are often considered a good way to get people to talk in more depth than they do in questionnaires, but the researcher's personality, and way of communicating, can impact on the encounter. So, using interviews has pros and cons. Interviews are often still a good way to gather information, but the discussion of the study methods should explain whether the researcher thought about the problems with their chosen methods, and describe any ways in which they sought to reduce these. Where and when data were collected may also be relevant (Astin, 2009): if staff are interviewed after a night shift, they may feel disinclined to detailed discussions because all they would want to do is get to bed. If they are asked to interrupt a busy shift, they may not be well placed to enter into any depth of discussion. Some of these limitations may be unavoidable, but if the researcher has highlighted and considered them, then there is a better chance that they tried to overcome them.

So, when you look at methods, you are really checking: how the information was gathered, whether this was a good way of gathering it, whether the way in which data were gathered was likely to mean that the information the researchers said they were looking for was found, and if anything in the methods was likely to mean that the apparent findings were actually influenced by other things (biases and confounding variables). Someone opining that the noise in ICU was not an issue because they wanted to get home to bed rather than because they really did not think it was an issue would fall into the final category.

Sampling

Sampling is about who or what was included in the study. The sample influences the quality of a study, but the question is not so much 'Is the sample big enough?' as 'Is the sample appropriate?' The issue is this: is it likely that the right type and quality of data would have been gathered using this sample? If a qualitative study used interviews to gain an in-depth understanding of patients' experiences of noise on ICU, a sample of 100 participants might be worrying. Unless there was a fairly big research team, the interviews might not have been conducted in much depth, and thus good quality data might not have been gathered, even though the sample was 'big'. Because it is depth of information, not generalizability, that is sought, qualitative research typically uses small numbers of participants (McGrath and Johnson, 2003), and gathers information until what is termed 'data saturation', where no new information or insights are coming to light, is achieved (see Chapter 6). Ten participants might have been a better number in qualitative enquiry, because this would allow the interviewer to explore each individual's experience in some depth. On the other hand, if the research fell within the quantitative paradigm and used a questionnaire with yes/no answers to identify whether or not staff thought noise in ICU mattered, then 100 or more staff would probably be a good sample size, and 10 way too few to do any very meaningful statistical analysis. So, size alone is not the issue. It depends on what size you need to do what you need to do.

As well as the numbers involved, the sample should tell you the characteristics of the people or places involved. If Konrad reads a study in which the 'sample' was 20 ICU staff, the details of the sample should include whether they were nurses, medical staff, physiotherapists, technicians or a mix of all staff, as well as how many there were. This means that he can see exactly what was studied, and who the results should apply to. How the researchers decided who or what to include in the sample is usually achieved by using inclusion and exclusion criteria: criteria which say who or what could be invited to be in the study and who or what could not (Coughlan, Cronin and Ryan, 2007). If Konrad finds a study of staff's views on noise in ICU whose inclusion criteria were nursing staff who had been qualified more than 6 months, and exclusion criteria as staff other than nurses and nurses of Band 7 or above, it is clear who the results apply to: nurses who have been qualified more than 6 months but who are employed on Band 6 or below.

The way in which the participants were selected also matters (Coughlan, Cronin and Ryan, 2007). Like just about everything else, the best way to do this depends on the type of research. Quantitative research aims to produce generalizable results; so the sample should be selected in a way that makes this possible, often by using what is known as probability sampling and randomly selecting people from a population. Qualitative research, in contrast, does not aim to achieve generalizability. Rather than using randomization, it is often necessary to seek out people who are particularly knowledgeable or have specific experiences related to the subject in question because they are the most likely to provide the depth of insight required. So, the 'best' way to sample depends on the aim of the study, and the methodology. Some sampling methods include

Probability sampling

Probability sampling is often considered the best method of sampling in quantitative research. It is essentially random sampling, in which everyone in the target population has an equal chance of being selected for the research, so that the results are equally likely to apply to anyone in that population. A sampling frame, such as a list of everyone in the population is used, and from this individuals are randomly selected.

Randomization can be carried out in various ways, depending on the subject and available sample: these include simple random sampling, stratified random sampling, systematic random sampling and cluster random sampling.

Non-probability sampling

Non-probability sampling is not generally seen as being as good as probability sampling for quantitative research. However it is usually superior to probability sampling for qualitative enquiry. Examples of non-probability sampling are:

Purposive sampling: the research subjects are selected on purpose because they are thought likely to provide the most comprehensive data for the matter under investigation. This can be a very valuable approach in qualitative research, for example, when people need to be selected because they are likely to be able to give deep or unique insights into a subject (Astin, 2009; McGrath and Johnson, 2003). However, it is less useful in quantitative enquiry, where the aim is to produce generalizable results.

Snowball sampling: the initial research subject or subjects refer the researcher to other potential participants (Parahoo, 2006). This can be useful in qualitative enquiry when the researcher is trying to find people who have particular experiences or views, and other participants may know who they are and can point the researcher to them, especially when they are difficult to access or identify by other means.

Convenience sampling: the sample is made up of the people who are available or accessible at the time. In quantitative research it creates the problem that the whole population do not have the chance to be selected, so the sample is unlikely to be representative of the population as a whole. In qualitative research, it means that these may not be the best people to involve; they are just the ones who could be accessed at the time. Although this approach to sampling may seem quite random, it is not random in research terms, because the whole population is not available or known, and there is not an equal chance of everyone from the population being included in the research.

Volunteer sampling: this is a self-selecting sample; those who volunteer participate. It is unlikely to be a representative sample of the population as a whole, and may not mean that the people with the most relevant experiences volunteer.

Although certain samples are the ideal in certain situations, it is not always possible to get the ideal. The ideal for study that explores people's recollections of noise in ICU might be to use a purposive sample of people who were known to have been in an ICU at a particularly noisy time; but this is unlikely to be possible. Instead, a volunteer sample of all ex-ICU patients might be used. This it is perfectly acceptable, and probably the most pragmatic approach. It has limitations, but does not stop the research from being usable.

In some cases a large enough sample is recruited, but not all of those who were recruited participate. In cases where recruitment does not guarantee participation (for example, where a questionnaire is sent to a list of people), and where numbers matter, usually at least 50 per cent participation or a 50 per cent response rate is needed for the results to be considered valid (Polit and Beck, 2006). If Konrad finds a study in which a questionnaire was distributed to all the staff on a unit, and whose results showed that they were all very concerned about noise, that might seem very convincing. However, if the response rate was 25 per cent, this apparent finding would be questionable. The reason for 75 % of the staff not responding is unknown. It might mean that they all felt ambivalent about noise, so the high agreement from those who responded does not really mean that there is broad support for reducing noise.

Ethical considerations

The principles of research ethics in healthcare are not really any different from any other branch of the ethics of healthcare: they concern doing good (beneficence), doing no harm (non-maleficence), respecting autonomy and seeking justice (Beauchamp and Childress, 2001). The main consideration in research ethics is whether the research in question fulfils these criteria. However, there are very few situations in life where it is possible to do good to everyone, no harm to anyone, respect every aspect of autonomy and be completely fair. Even if the only possible harm from a piece of research is that people who agree to participate in interviews will give up some of their time and maybe feel nervous about the interview, it is a potential harm. All research should be ethically sound, but balancing benefit and harm and drawing the acceptable line for what is ethical and what is not is not always easy.

In terms of harm, the question is whether study participants are subjected to any actual or potential physical harm, discomfort or psychological distress (Coughlan, Cronin and Ryan, 2007). If they are, then whether they were aware of this, gave informed consent knowing this, whether the researchers took appropriate steps to minimize the risk of harm, whether the nature of the harm was deemed to be acceptable and whether the benefits to individuals or society outweighed the potential cost to the participants are usually considered. It may be deemed acceptable for there to be a risk of participants being embarrassed or upset during interviews, provided they are aware of this risk, the researcher makes efforts to minimize the risk and measures are put in place to support participants who experience these feelings (Whiting, 2008).

Another common consideration in research ethics relates to autonomy and concerns participants giving informed consent (Coughlan, Cronin and Ryan, 2007). Informed consent means that participants understand the study's purpose, what is required of them, what the risks and benefits of participating are and how the results will be used. The need for informed consent applies to whoever is involved in a study regardless of whether they are members of staff, patients, relatives of patients, healthy volunteers etc. Consent should also be a reversible process, insofar as participants should have the right to withdraw from a study at any time without fear of reprisals, or coercion to continue to participate. There are sometimes reasons why informed consent is not gained, and, very occasionally, this is justifiable, but the reason for such a decision has to be very clear and convincing. There are also special considerations where the participants are deemed to have specific vulnerabilities (for example, where they are minors, or have learning disabilities). However, the basic principle is that informed consent to participate in research has to be sought from the appropriate party or parties.

Consent to participate in research should be gained without coercion: which includes the use of status, power or incentives to try to persuade individuals to participate against their will. Incentives are not necessarily wrong: it depends upon whether they are used to coerce individuals to participate with a fear of reprisals if they do not, or whether participants can anonymously weigh up the potential benefits of incentives as part of the informed consent process. Drugs trials are often conducted on healthy volunteers who answer advertisements offering payment for their participation: they are not personally coerced to participate even though they receive financial recompense. On the other hand, if you are approached by the person who is doing the Christmas rota and asked to participate in an interview for their research if you want to see your family at all over the festive season, that is coercion.

The requirement to respect autonomy includes considering whether participants' identity is kept confidential or anonymized (Coughlan, Cronin and Ryan, 2007). Confidentiality means that individual identities are not linked to any information provided, and that these identities are never publicly divulged (Polit and Beck, 2006). Anonymity means that no one knows who the participants are, and that their identity cannot be linked to the data even by the researcher (Burns and Grove, 2005). Face-to-face interviews never achieve anonymity in this sense because the researcher would know who the participants are. Even if the data generated from conversations with them is immediately coded as 'participant 1' on all notes, transcripts and analytical processes, the researcher knows who participant 1 is and has met them. This does not make the interview unethical, but the participants should be clear about who will and will not know their true identity and exactly what they are being offered: confidentiality or anonymity. Participants should also know what will happen to the data that they provide, because if it is published, even when their real names are not used, they might be recognizable, for instance by the use of quotes from interview transcripts. A member of staff in an ICU might carry out a study on her own unit in which she interviews colleagues about noise levels. When the study is published, other staff in the unit would very likely be able to recognize individuals from the quotes, even if their names are not used.

It is unlikely that a research report in a journal will be able to delve into all the intricacies of these points. It is a good idea to see whether a study that you read about was approved and monitored by an ethics committee or ethics review board (Coughlan, Cronin and Ryan, 2007). Having a study approved by an ethics committee means that the ethical considerations were debated by a group whose role it is to weigh up all the ethical concerns, in more depth than a journal article can allow for the reporting of. If a report you read is actually audit or clinical evaluation, it may not have required ethics committee approval, but it may have local governance committee approval or something similar. As Chapter 2 discussed, the divisions between research, audit and clinical evaluation are not always clear cut, and ethical principles should apply to all practice, not just research; so audit or evaluation should also fulfil the ethical obligations of healthcare (Wade, 2005). However, it will probably not have the same body approving it as research does.

Analysis

A very important part of deciding whether or not to use the findings presented in a research report is whether the information gathered was analysed appropriately. If it was not, then however diligently it was gathered, the results will be flawed and the conclusions and recommendations probably not worth acting on. The first thing is to check if the data was analysed in the right sort of way (qualitative data analysed using qualitative processes; quantitative data using quantitative processes). If Konrad finds a qualitative study, using interviews with ICU staff as the research method, he would expect the method of data analysis to be something which looked at understanding the meaning of what was said. This could be done by dividing the interview transcripts into codes and then combining the codes which were similar into categories, rather than statistical tests or tables of results. On the other hand if he reads a report in which quantitative data were gathered, he would expect numerical or statistical tests to be used for data analysis. The next consideration is this: was the specific type of analysis used correct? For example, were the right statistical tests used (Coughlan, Cronin and Ryan, 2007)? The processes of analysing quantitative and qualitative data are discussed in Chapters 5 and 6, but the right things should have been done with the data for the results to be meaningful.

Reliability and validity

Reliability and validity are concerned with whether the apparent findings from a study are really true.

Reliability is about whether a particular test, procedure or tool will produce similar results in different circumstances, assuming nothing else has changed: will it reliably measure whatever it is meant to be measuring (Roberts and Priest, 2006)? Validity refers to how close what we think we are measuring is to what we are actually measuring (Roberts and Priest, 2006). In quantitative research, statisticians have devised procedures for estimating the reliability and validity of various research processes (Roberts and Priest, 2006). It is immediately clear that these will not work in qualitative research, because no mathematics or statistics are involved. Some of the concepts associated with reliability and validity are also unacceptable to many qualitative researchers, because qualitative research acknowledges that things like feelings or responses to experiences can be transient and that all experience is highly individual and circumstantial. Some criteria have nonetheless been developed to demonstrate the quality of qualitative research, and the terms reliability and validity are often replaced by the concept of trustworthiness (Lincoln and Guba, 1985). However, it is also argued that the range of qualitative methodologies that exist makes it impossible to give a one-size-fits-all-way of demonstrating quality qualitative research (Jootun and McGhee, 2009). This is debated in more detail in Chapter 6, but what is important, in principle, in evaluating any study is to check that it was conducted systematically and robustly.

Results and findings

In order to use the findings from a study, you need to know what they were. If you want to use research in practice, rather than write an assignment critiquing a piece of research, you do not necessarily need to worry greatly about how well presented the results are. Nevertheless, if they are not very clear, you may get bored or confused trying to read them and you may (wrongly) assume that it is you who does not understand and might jump to the conclusions and recommendations section and assume that what the study says you should do is right. If that is the case, then you should probably not use the study to change practice. You need to read the results/ findings and conclusions, to make sure that what the researcher recommends matches what they found.

Often studies present the findings and then (or in combination) a discussion of these, which explains and explores them and their implications, and links them with what was already known on the subject. You need to read both sections to feel confident to use (or decide not to use) the findings from a piece of research, because the discussion will often explain the results and why the researcher interpreted them in the way they did in more detail than the findings or results section does.

If you cannot make sense of the results, the chances are you should not use that particular piece of research.

Conclusions and recommendations

The conclusions and recommendations made in a study should be clearly linked to the findings. If Konrad reads a study whose results show that the most noise in ICUs occurs during new admissions in the daytime, he might be surprised if the recommendations are to try to decrease noise at night. That might still be a sensible thing to do, because the night is when everybody should be asleep, but that is not what the study's results show.

The conclusions and recommendations should also fit the paradigm or methodology in question. If Konrad reads a qualitative study exploring whether or not newly qualified nurses are aware of noise on ICU, it would not be possible for it to give concrete recommendations that would definitely reduce noise by a certain amount. It could give plenty of ideas for practice development, but because the study did not aim to prove anything, it could not guarantee specific outcomes. However, if he reads a quantitative study which shows beyond reasonable doubt that having a different type of waste bin reduces noise, the study might be able, with some confidence, to recommend which was the best bin for every ICU.

Is the study is applicable?

An important part of using research in practice is to decide whether a study is applicable to your area of practice. This is about looking at exactly where and with whom the research was carried out, and deciding how far that group might match where you want to use the results. The report should give you enough information to think about whether to use it exactly as it stands, whether to proceed but with caution, juggling a few bits because the setting was not quite the same or whether it was so different that you cannot possibly use it.

Using existing frameworks to evaluate research

Remembering everything that you need to look at to check a study's quality can be quite demanding, and you may have better things to remember, so it can be useful to have a tool to guide you and make sure that you do not miss anything. There are several existing tools which you can use. One such set of tools are the Critical Appraisal Skills Programme (CASP project) tools, which are available at www.sph.nhs.uk/what-we-do/public-health-workforce/resources/critical-appraisals-skills-programme (accessed 1 February 2011)

There is also a brief outline of things you might want to consider in evaluating studies for use in practice in Appendix 1. Some of the points in it are discussed in detail in Chapters 5, 6 and 7. The important thing is to use a tool which is suitable for the type of study you are looking at, and which you understand and feel comfortable with. A tool is meant to help you, not become a further complication to using research, so you should not feel obliged to use something that does not work for you. You also need to use the tool bearing in mind that your agenda is whether or not to use the piece of research in practice. Although a checklist might ask things like, 'Is the review of the literature good?' and even if you answer with a 'no', if the rest of the paper is very clear, focused and does all the right things, you might well want to use the findings. Similarly, if a question asks: 'Are the results clearly presented?' and the answer is 'no', but you spend an hour figuring them out and realize that although the writer's style was hard to understand, the results seem accurate and very useful, then you should probably consider using them.

Summary

The aim of evaluating research in order to decide whether or not to use it in practice is to see whether a study looked at what it said it did, whether the way in which information was gathered and analysed was appropriate and systematic, whether reasonable ethical standards were maintained, if the results and conclusions seem to fit the findings, and whether this is relevant to your practice. Precisely how all this is achieved in quantitative, qualitative and mixed methods research is discussed in more detail in the next three chapters.

Worked example

Honour works as a community nurse, in an area which has a relatively high population of older people. She has noticed that, in many cases, their families provide a great deal of care that individuals with dementia need, but that they do not necessarily have a great deal of support themselves. She wants to develop services for such families, and has looked for research on directions she might take. Two of the papers which she has found are

Paper 1

Title: Living with dementia: carers' perspectives

Study aim: To explore the experiences of people who care for a parent who has dementia.

Methodology: The paper describes itself as using 'a hermeneutic, phenomenological approach to explore the lived experiences of adults who care for a parent who has dementia'.

Methods: The methods are described as 'in-depth interviews with carers, in which the researcher allowed the participant to lead in describing their experiences of caring for their mother or father'. Each participant was interviewed twice, the second interview being an opportunity to build on the first. Each interview lasted approximately one hour. The interviews were recorded and transcribed verbatim. The researcher used a field journal to record additional data about the interviews and their own feelings about and inputs into the interactions.

Sample: Five women participated in the interviews. All participants lived near, but in a separate house from, their parent(s). Their parent(s) lived alone or with an elderly partner. The study was conducted in England. A letter was sent to people who were known to care for a parent who had dementia, inviting them to participate.

Ethics approval: Approval from an NHS Research Ethics committee was obtained. Informed consent was obtained from all participants.

Data analysis: The interviews and journal entries were analysed using thematicanalysis. The researcher carried out all the analysis.

Findings: Key themes were presented as: Hidden work, no time off, emotional demands, conflicting demands, employment, short break care, understanding and support, service provision. These were supported by quotes to explain and illustrate the points made. Transcripts were anonymized, but the quotes were used which were attributed to all five participants.

Conclusions: Adults who provide care for a parent with dementia felt that their workload was poorly acknowledged. They had very little time off, and short break care mainly involved admission to a nursing home. Juggling the carers' own home demands and those of their parent(s) was very difficult, carers often felt exhausted, with little prospect of rest. 'Fighting for services' was an additional demand, alongside the frustration and time taken to organize and maintain services, and the feeling that their contribution was not acknowledged or valued by service providers. Their work was emotionally draining, and even when physical care was not required, they were constantly 'on call', and worried about their parents' safety and well-being. This could affect their own health and employment (they became 'unreliable employees' due to their parents' fluctuating needs). In addition, their dual role as child and carer could be distressing.

Evaluation

Subject: The subject seems relevant, and the title reflects what the paper is about.

Methodology: Hermeneutic phenomenology is a qualitative methodology, and qualitative methodology is appropriate for in depth exploration of individuals' experiences.

Methods: In-depth interviews are an appropriate method for qualitative research and for this subject. Participants led the interviews, so it was likely that what mattered most to them was discussed. This might mean that everyone was not asked or did not discuss exactly the same things, but in qualitative research the aim is that all relevant and potentially very individual data are gathered. Subjective and individual experiences are the focus, so flexibility on exactly what is asked and discussed is necessary. Conducting two interviews with each participant would have created an opportunity to develop and build on data, and may well have generated greater depth of data than one interview would have. Whether the interviews were structured, semi-structured or unstructured is not discussed, but they were clearly not highly and inflexibly structured, because they moved with the priorities of the participants. They were probably semi-structured or unstructured, both of which fit a qualitative methodology.

The location of the interviews was not stated, and might have had an effect on the data, for example, if they were conducted in participant's homes, this might have meant that individuals were less inconvenienced, more relaxed and that any perceived power relationship between researcher and participant was reduced.

The researcher attempted to address their own effect on data by using and analysing a field journal, which is a commonly used method in qualitative research (discussed in more detail in Chapter 6).

Sample: The study had a small number of participants, which is appropriate for this methodology as it allows depth of data to be gathered. All the participants were female, and although this limits the contexts to which the study might be applied, as long as this is noted, it is not a problem in using the information from the study in developing practice. A volunteer sample seems to have been used: everyone on a list of people known to care for a parent who had dementia was invited (how this list was generated is not clear), and individuals who volunteered participated. This might have meant that people with particular insights or experiences were not involved, because they did not volunteer, but this sample would still have provided useful insights, as those who volunteered are likely to have been interested in the subject and had information to offer.

Ethical approval: Ethics committee approval was obtained and the report stated that informed consent was gained from participants, and that they were assured of confidentiality of information. Whether or not participants were aware that they could withdraw from the study was not clear and whether they were aware of how findings might be used is not mentioned.

Data analysis: Thematic analysis seems an appropriate approach and is a recognized method of analysing qualitative data (see Chapter 6).

Findings: The findings were presented under the subheadings of the themes developed. Exactly how the themes were developed was not discussed, but the quotes used seemed to correspond with the meaning of the themes that they were linked to. Quotes from all the participants were used, suggesting that the range of views expressed were noted by the researcher.

Conclusions: The conclusions relate to the findings. No specific recommendations for practice were made.

This study would probably provide useful ideas for Honour to consider in developing services. Although no specific recommendations were made, the insights offered are likely to provide her with ideas which could be developed. The intention of qualitative enquiry is not to produce precisely generalizable findings but to provide insight and understanding, to guide practice. This paper could be used in this way.

Paper 2

Title: Stressors in dementia care

Study aim: The aim of this study was to determine what causes stress for people who care for a relative who has dementia.

Methodology: This was not stated.

Methods: The study used a questionnaire to identify the factors which create stress for people who care for a relative who has dementia. The questionnaire was designed by a group of three community nurses who were developing a dementia care service, and piloted with two carers. The questionnaire had two sections. One related to things which might cause stress for carers, and one to things which might reduce stress. Each used a four-point scale against which respondents were asked to rate their views. In section one they were asked to rate items as being: very stressful, stressful, neutral or not stressful and section two as items potentially reducing stress: significantly, slightly, not at all or creating more stress. The questionnaire contained 30 items, 15 in each section.

Sample: The questionnaire was sent to 57 people who were known to care for relatives who had dementia. How their names and contact details were known was not clear. The study was carried out in a large city in the UK. A response rate of 80 per cent was achieved.

Ethical approval: The study did not mention whether ethical approval was granted. It was described as a part of an ongoing service development project.

Data analysis: This was not discussed.

Results: The results were presented as mean scores for each item on the questionnaire. The highest scoring stressors were (mean scores in brackets, from maximum score of 4, 4 being the most stressful): Conflicting advice or information (3.6), Liaising with health and social care services (3.5), Worrying about relatives' safety (3.4), Constant demands (3.3) and Financial concerns (3.0). The items which scored highest for reducing stress were Keyworker to act as central liaison point (3.2), 'Sitter' services on a reliable and planned basis (3.1), Financial advice (3.0) and Reliable short break services (2.7).

Conclusions and recommendations: The conclusions seemed to echo the results, outlining the most important areas for developing support in light of the findings, and stating that this was the next stage of the service development project.

Evaluation

Title: The title and aim suggest that this study could be relevant for Honour. The title matches what the study is about.

Methodology: The methodology is not stated. Because it was a part of a larger service development project, it may not have been regarded primarily as research (which may also explain the lack of ethics committee approval). The way in which data were generated and analysed match a quantitative paradigm, and this approach is consistently used. The lack of statement of methodology alone does not mean the study should be disregarded provided that it follows a logical and consistent format.

Methods: A questionnaire was a suitable way of ascertaining the views of this population. It would not give any depth of understanding of individuals' experiences, but could be useful to highlight broad areas in which services could be improved or developed.

The study pre-specified what was being explored in terms of stressors, with no option for respondents adding further information, so any issues which might create or reduce stress that the study team did not think of would not have been included. There was no suggestion that the items on the scales were derived from previous studies or literature, and service users did not seem to be involved in developing the questionnaire, so some key issues may have been omitted. However, the questionnaire was developed by three experts in the field and piloted with two service users, which means that there was some agreement that the items were a valid way to assess stressors and that nothing major was missed out. Whether everyone would interpret the statements made on the questionnaire in the same way might be questionable, but this may have been overcome to some extent by piloting the tool.

Rating scales can be problematic in creating an 'extreme response' bias (i.e., people naturally veer towards responding at one end of the scale or the other, not the mid points), and acquiescence bias (where people tend towards agreeing with the statement made). However, they can also be useful for gauging the overall views of a population.

Sample: The sample was relatively small for this type of study, but it was perhaps the largest available for this project, possibly the number available to a particular service.

What type of sampling was used, and how those to whom the questionnaire was sent were identified was not stated. It may well have been the total local population or the known local population, or a convenience sample. The lack of clear sampling framework does not mean the study is not usable, but it does affect its generalizability. The high response rate means that there is relatively little missing data, and might indicate that the population studied considered this an important subject. However, it could also indicate they felt obliged to respond, particularly if they used the service in question, and this might bring into question whether this feeling of obligation affected other responses.

Data analysis: The data analysis process was not discussed, but uses descriptive statistics (see Chapter 5): while this limits how far the results can be generalized, it is appropriate for the sample size and study design (the study seems to be intended primarily to direct local practice development). Whether a mean value should be used for rating scales is debatable. Chapter 5 discusses this in more detail, but usually ordinal data (data that are ordered, but have values which may not necessarily be equidistant from each other, such as satisfaction scales rated 1–4) or nominal (data which are given a name but which have no numerical value) should not be presented using a mean value. This is because, for instance, in this case, the 'average' of stressful and very stressful does not exist in the way that the average of the actual numbers 4 and 3 does. Some people argue that using mean scores for such scales is acceptable, and some that it is not (Blaikie, 2003; Jamieson, 2004). Generally speaking, caution should be exercised in relying on the precise accuracy of results where findings from ordinal rating scales are presented as mean values. This does not preclude the study findings being considered in Honour's practice development, particularly if the scores are designed to show trends not exact measures, but reliance on their precision should be avoided.

Findings: The findings clearly state what people who care for a relative who has dementia found stressful, what was helpful and gave an idea of how important each issue or factor was.

Conclusions: The conclusions and recommendations match the results and indicate how these will be used to develop local practice. There is no claim that the findings from this study are generalizable beyond local practice.

Overall, although the paper has limitations, there is nothing intrinsically wrong with it. The study does not claim that it's findings are generalizable: they seem to be designed to develop local practice, and should be seen in this context. Whether the study was intended as 'research' or 'service evaluation' or 'service development' (see Chapter 2) is not clear, but the important issue is perhaps more the quality of the information than its label. It would be useful for giving Honour ideas about developing practice and, as it was part of a larger service development project, it might be useful for her to contact the team concerned and discuss possibilities for her own service development with them.

Seen jointly, the two papers have some common findings which may give Honour a better indication of the importance of these than just one study would.

Appraising quantitative research 5

The principles of quantitative enquiry

The other day, there was an announcement to the effect that 94 per cent of the population were worried about the current financial situation in Britain. No one had asked me though, and I am a member of the population, so how could this be accurate?

The intention of quantitative enquiry is to produce evidence which can be applied to whole populations, but usually all the members of a population cannot actually be studied. A sample of the population is therefore used and statistical tests applied to the data gathered to make predictions about whether it would apply to the population as a whole (Thomas, 2005; Windish and Diener-West, 2006). That is why it was probably OK to announce the views of the nation without getting my opinion first.

Practice situations in which quantitative enquiry is likely to be useful

Quantitative enquiry is useful where the intention is to discover, with a reasonable degree of certainty, whether or not something is likely to be apply to a whole population (Thomas, 2005; Windish and Diener-West, 2006). It is often used to test new drugs, interventions, screening processes and assessment processes. It might be a useful approach for the type of information that Jo is looking for, because she wants to find an assessment tool which any member of staff can pick up and use for anyone who is admitted to her unit regardless of who they are, or why they are being admitted.

Research question/hypothesis

Quantitative research often (but not always) uses a hypothesis. A hypothesis is a statement about the association between variables, which is either upheld or not depending on the results of the study (Parahoo, 2006). A hypothesis might state, 'Tool A improves the assessment of the emotional state of teenagers.' So there is a statement of association between the use of tool A and the assessment of teenagers' emotional state. Depending on what the study shows, the hypothesis is either upheld or not. Hypotheses are upheld, not proved, because every single person in the population and every possible eventuality are not usually accounted for (for example, the omission of my valuable opinion on the state of the nation's finances).

Usually a study with a hypothesis will in fact have two hypotheses: an Alternate Hypothesis (usually just called the hypothesis) and a Null Hypothesis. The two concern the same thing, but the hypothesis is a statement of association or effect and the null hypothesis is a statement of no effect or no association (Ren 2009; Thomas, 2005; Windish and Diener-West, 2006). Jo might look at a paper with the null hypothesis: 'Tool A does not affect the assessment of the emotional state of teenagers' (no association between tool A and improved assessment). The corresponding hypothesis would be: 'Tool A improves the assessment of the emotional state of teenagers' (association between tool A and improved assessment).

Usually, both hypotheses are needed because the way statistical tests work is that a hypothesis can only be upheld by refuting the null hypothesis (Ren, 2009). So it is really the null hypothesis that is tested and upheld or not, and, by association, the hypothesis (which is its direct opposite) is either upheld or not.

Many quantitative studies have hypotheses, and experimental studies usually have them, but not all quantitative studies need to or should. Studies which do not aim to show the cause and effect between variables or to demonstrate something beyond reasonable doubt may instead refer to the purpose of the study, the research problem or question. Jo might find a study about whether staff found a particular assessment tool useful. This would probably not have a hypothesis because there was no intention to show a relationship between two variables. It might nonetheless involve quantification of what large numbers of practitioners found useful or not useful about the tool.

The thing to check is whether the study has a clear and appropriate statement regarding the intention of the research, and, if it has a hypothesis, whether it has a corresponding null hypothesis which is the exact opposite. (Although some study reports only state the hypothesis, even when a null hypothesis was also used, so if the null hypothesis is not mentioned, it is not always a reason to disregard a study.)

Research design/methodology

Most quantitative studies fall within two broad designs: experimental and observational (also called descriptive) (Windish and Diener-West, 2006).

Experimental studies

In experimental studies, it is no surprise to hear, an experiment of some kind is set up. The experiment should be designed to test a particular thing and to isolate that from other factors, so that it is quite certain that any effect seen is to the result of whatever is being tested, not something else. Experiments almost always need a hypothesis and null hypothesis because the researcher is trying to show whether there is an association between what is being tested and some kind of outcome. Experiments can be set up in many ways: laboratory work, administration of drugs or other interventions, testing new assessment tools (which Jo might be interested in) and a whole range of other things.

Experiments may include a control group (a group which either has no intervention at all, or the intervention they would have had if the experiment was not happening) (Parahoo, 2006). Jo might find an experiment in which young people in a control group were assessed without using any tool, while the experimental group were assessed using a tool. Ideally, the control and intervention groups should be as exact a match as possible in terms of key factors such as age, sex and diagnosis. This reduces the chance of any apparent differences in the results from each group because of the characteristics of the individuals within the groups, rather than the intervention being tested (Parahoo, 2006). In a study comparing adolescents who were assessed using a new tool with those assessed using no tool, where those in the first group were male and those in the second female, any apparent effect from using the tool might actually be because the people in that group were male, rather than anything to do with the tool.

Where an intervention and control group is used, the ideal way of deciding who goes into each group is random allocation of participants to one group or another (Parahoo, 2006). This means that there is an equal chance of every person who is in the study being placed in either group. In an experimental study comparing the effect of using an assessment tool against using no tool, the research subjects might be randomly allocated into groups who were or were not assessed using the tool. The method of randomization could be that the first person admitted to a unit would be in the control group, the second in the intervention group, the third in the control group, etc. While the third person would always go into the control group, nothing about them except the fact that they were the third to arrive places them in this group. If they had arrived an hour earlier and been admitted to number two, they would have been in the intervention group.

If the researcher selects who will go into each group, there is the potential for the selection to be biased, for example, 'difficult' cases or ones which they feel would benefit from the new assessment tool might be placed in the intervention group. If allocation is randomized, this possibility is avoided. This increases the chance that if something appears to happen to those who are assessed using the tool, it is because of the assessment tool, not because the people in that group were handpicked as those most likely to benefit, or some other reason.

A common example of an experimental study is a Randomized controlled trial (RCT): a study where people are randomly allocated to receive (or not receive) a particular intervention. The controlled element is because as well as the intervention group (who receive the intervention being tested) there is a comparison (control) group which receives a placebo, another treatment or no treatment at all.

Sometimes the term 'blinding' is used in experiments. A blind trial means that the research participants do not know which study group they are in (for example, whether they receive a new drug or a placebo). This may increase the accuracy of the results by removing the chance of any apparent effects being due to a person knowing that they were or were not receiving a drug, such as the 'feel good factor' of believing one is receiving treatment (Lee, 2006a). Single blinding is when the research participant does not know which group they are in, but the researcher knows which person has which intervention. This means that they could treat participants differently, or to hint to them about the group they are in, which might influence the outcome of the study. To overcome this, double blinding may be used, in which neither the researcher nor the person involved in the experiment knows whether they are in the experimental or control group. However, double blinding is often difficult to achieve. In a study Jo reads, a group of young people might have been randomly allocated to being assessed using a tool or not using a tool. Blinding in this study might have been problematic, because the young people could be aware of how they were assessed. The staff admitting young people would know whether or not they were using an assessment tool for each individual, so double blinding would almost certainly have been impossible.

When you decide whether or not to use the results of an experimental study, the key factors are whether the experiment was likely to effectively test what it said it would, or to compare what it said it would; whether any comparison groups were randomized from the same population; and whether blinding was used (if possible and appropriate). You should look for what would be a reasonable expectation: it would be misguided not to use evidence from an RCT simply because blinding was not used, when blinding would have been impossible.

Observational or descriptive studies

There are many things which are best studied using a quantitative approach but which are not suitable for an experimental design. Quantitative studies that are not experimental are usually called observational or descriptive studies. In these studies, no attempt is made to change the conditions which exist (Russell, 2005). The drugs which people receive are not changed, the assessment tools used when admitting them are not changed; what is already happening is studied. The results cannot usually be as confidently generalized to whole populations as those from experimental studies, because they are more likely to be affected by the characteristics of the people or groups of people involved.

Some examples of designs for descriptive or observational studies are

Case-control studies

In case-control studies, sometimes also referred to as quasi-experimental studies (Abbott and Sapsford, 1998), individuals receive an intervention of interest or have developed the disease or condition of interest (cases), and controls are then found based on who matches the cases for key characteristics (such as diagnosis, age and sex), as far as possible and who did not receive the intervention or develop the disease or condition (Zondervan, Cardon and Kennedy, 2002). Jo might find a case-control study in which young people who were assessed using a certain tool (cases) were compared to controls who closely matched these young people in terms of diagnosis, age and gender, but who were not assessed using that tool. In case-control studies it is more important to have a close match between the cases and controls than for them to be representative of the population in question.

Longitudinal studies

In longitudinal studies, individuals who have something of interest to the researcher are followed over time: possibly for months or years (Parahoo, 2006). A longitudinal study of an assessment tool for young people with mental health problems might study how the first 100 young people who were assessed using a particular tool fared over the subsequent year, with particular interest in how the initial assessment seemed to influence this.

Cross-sectional Studies

Cross-sectional studies are carried out at one point in time and provide a 'snap-shot' of whatever is of interest (Abbott and Sapsford, 1998), for example, disease characteristics at a given point in time, or the views of a population at one point in time. Jo might find a cross-sectional study of what all the staff working on a unit during January thought of an assessment tool which had been introduced three months previously. It would provide a snapshot of what a range of staff thought at that time and might allow comparisons between what nurses, support workers and psychiatrists thought of the tool.

Prospective/retrospective

A prospective study is one that is planned so as to gather data in the future, for example, after the introduction of a new assessment tool. A retrospective study is one that relies on data that have already been collected (for example, through medical records) (Parahoo, 2006).

Although certain study designs are sometimes described as 'better' than others (for example, an RCT is often regarded as the highest form of evidence), what really matters is whether the study design was appropriate for the subject, and whether the overall quality of the study was good: a good-quality case-control study may be much better and more worthy of attention than a poor quality RCT, even though an RCT is theoretically the 'better' method. You should also consider the fitness for purpose of the study. If the intervention that you are giving is a new drug, you might want to be sure, beyond reasonable doubt, that you can safely give it to more or less anyone, so a high-quality RCT might be the only thing you would accept. However, if you are looking for research about whether or not parents think that it would be useful to have a vending machine near the ward their child is on, you might feel able to proceed on less definite evidence. Both matter of course, but installing a vending machine is a less risky thing to do than administering new drugs across a population.

Sampling

The various ways of selecting a sample and their merits were described in Chapter 4. The main things to consider in quantitative research are the following: how was the sample chosen? Was this right for the task? Were the right things/people sampled? Was the sample the right size for the task? And if it involved people responding, did enough respond? Although probability (random) sampling is often seen as the best approach for quantitative research, sometimes it cannot be achieved or is inappropriate: in a case-control study the controls cannot be randomly selected because they have to be matched to the cases. Often it might be ideal, but impractical, to use a random sample, particularly in descriptive studies. So, the question is: was the right or best possible sampling method used for the study in question? If it was not the best possible sample, what would the effect of this have been (for instance, does it invalidate the study, or just mean that it cannot be so confidently generalized)?

In quantitative enquiry, numbers matter. The intention is to be fairly sure that the findings from a study were not just due to chance, so enough participants are needed to achieve this. Researchers can use a sample size formula (such as the power calculation described later in the chapter) to find out the ideal number of participants needed to achieve this. It is useful if a paper reports on this because 'how big is big enough' really depends on what the study design and intention are, and what statistical tests are being used.

Methods of data collection

Quantitative research can use a whole range of data collection methods: measuring physiological parameters, interviews, questionnaires, attitude scales or observation tools, to name just a few. Some of the tools may sound like ones which can also be used in qualitative work, and indeed they can. It is the type of tool, for example, the type of interview or questionnaire which makes it suitable for qualitative or quantitative data collection. Questionnaires that consist of closed questions with a choice of fixed answers are suitable for quantitative research. Similarly, interviews in which only a yes/no answer is required, and which are administered to a large number of people, can be used. The key question is: does the method that was used seem likely to accurately gather the right type of data? This really concerns the reliability and validity of the method, tools and procedures involved.

Reliability and validity

Reliability is about whether the research design and tools will accurately and consistently measure what they are supposed to measure, or study what they are supposed to study (Wood, Ross-Kerr and Brink, 2006). A part of the reliability of a questionnaire is whether the questions in it address the subject under investigation, and whether everyone would take them to mean the same thing. The reliability of a tool may have been established by it being tested in previous research or by it having become accepted as a standardized test or scale. If a researcher develops a new tool, they should explain how they checked if it was a true and accurate measure of what they wanted to measure, for example, by piloting it with an appropriate population. If the researcher adapted an existing instrument it in some way, they should say how they knew it was still appropriate for use in the new format or context (Polit and Beck, 2006).

Reliability is also about whether the apparent results from a study are due to whatever the research is about, rather than because of an error in some part of the research process. This is dealt with by using reliability scores. If a study about how many staff used a new assessment tool had a 90 per cent reliability score, it would mean that 90 per cent of the score almost certainly related to the number of staff who were using the tool while 10 per cent of the score was less certain and possibly due to errors in how recordings were made, stored or analysed. The 90 per cent is then expressed as a decimal, so a 0.9 reliability score means that 90 per cent of the apparent score is true and 10 per cent is possibly due to error. A reliability of 80–90 per cent is generally considered acceptable (Roberts and Priest, 2006).

Validity concerns whether the research tool measures what it is supposed to measure (Roberts and Priest, 2006). The two main subdivisions of validity – internal and external validity – are described below, but basically validity means 'do the data really mean what the findings say they mean?'

Internal validity looks at whether or not the apparent outcomes of the study are a valid interpretation of events (Roberts and Priest, 2006): whether there could have been reasons other than the issue being studied for the outcomes. Some ways that this can be addressed are:

- Reducing the risk of factors such as the individual characteristics of participants having an effect on the study outcomes, or the results simply being
  due to chance. Using a random sampling mechanism, having a close enough

match between any groups being compared, and having a large enough sample size can help to reduce this risk.

- Making sure that the tool measures what it is supposed to or gets the right type of information, for example, by designing a questionnaire using a comprehensive literature review to guide the content, and then conducting a pilot study. (Known as content validity, Roberts and Priest, 2006.)
- Comparing the tool to other similar validated measures of the same concept or phenomenon: this can only be done when other such measures exist. (Known as criterion validity, Maltby *et al.*, 2010; Parahoo, 2006.)
- Establishing whether the study shows evidence that it is measuring what it claims to measure. For example, if Jo found a study which claimed a new assessment tool was effective based on staff liking it and using it, it might simply mean that the paperwork was easy to complete, not that it facilitated an effective assessment. (Known as construct validity, Parahoo, 2006.)

External validity is about how far the study can be assumed to work 'externally': how confidently the findings can be applied to people and situations other than those in the study. This might include who or what comprised the sample, the inclusion and exclusion criteria, how research subjects or participants were selected and how many there were (Maltby, 2010; Roberts and Priest, 2006). The way in which data were analysed also affects how confidently the findings can be generalized to whole populations.

Data analysis

Quantitative data are analysed using statistical methods. A range of statistical tests exist, and the right one has to be used for the right thing. Which test is the right one depends on

The study design
The size of the sample(s)
How the data were distributed (what they would look like on a graph)
What type of data were used (e.g., nominal, ordinal, interval, ratio)
The purpose of the study, e.g., to compare two groups, measure the views of a single group etc.

(Windish and Diener-West, 2006)

There are two main divisions of statistical tests: parametric and non-parametric tests (Maltby *et al.*, 2010: 207) and data gathered in quantitative research are often described as either parametric or non-parametric.

Parametric tests are based upon the assumptions that

- The observations/ data collected are independent of all other observations or data
- The data follow a normal distribution curve (the distribution is referred to as 'normal' if the shape of the graph it would make is 'bell shaped', see Figure 5.1)

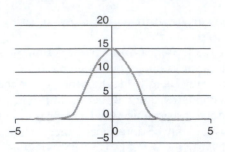

Figure 5.1   Diagram of a bell-shaped curve

- Interval data or ratio data are used. Both interval and ratio data are measured along a scale in which each position is the same distance from the next. For example, the difference between 1 mcg and 2 mcgs is the same as between 2 mcgs and 3 mcgs. The distinction is that in interval data an absolute zero score does not exist, whereas in ratio data it does.

(Maltby *et al.*, 2010: 179).

Non-parametric tests are usually used when:

- The data do not follow a normal distribution curve.
- Nominal or ordinal data are used. Nominal data are data which are differentiated by a system which has no numerical meaning, for example, a person's sex. Ordinal data are data that can be placed in order to show their relative position, for example, staff on Bands 1, 2, 3, 4, 5. However, unlike ratio or interval data there is not necessarily the same difference between each point on the scale (Maltby *et al.*, 2010: 180). There is not as much certainty that there is the same amount of difference between staff on Band 2 and Band 3 and staff on Band 3 and Band 4 as there is that the difference between 23 mcgs and 3–4 mcgs is the same amount.
- The sample size is small.

(Greenhalgh, 2010; Windish and Diener-West, 2006)

Non-parametric tests are generally less powerful than parametric tests (they are not as good at detecting small differences between groups). However, it is better to use a non-parametric test for non-parametric data than to use a parametric one on the wrong type of data.

There are usually viewed as being two levels of statistical analysis: descriptive statistics and inferential statistics.

Descriptive statistics

Descriptive statistics are used to summarize and display data using fairly basic calculations, usually the mean (the average: the sum of all the values in a set divided by the number of values), median (the value at the precise middle when all the values are arranged in numerical order) and the mode (value that occurs most frequently) are used (Thomas 2004). These are used to calculate what is known as the central tendency: the central value of the data (Windish and Diener-West, 2006).

Usually, mean scores should only be used for parametric data (interval or ratio data), because for an average to be calculated, there has to be the same distance between all the points studied. The mean dose from 1 mcg, 2 mcg, 4 mcg and 5 mcg could be calculated as 3 mcg. However, if a scale of 1–5 is used to measure staff confidence in using a new assessment tool with 1: not at all confident, 2: not confident, 3: uncertain of level of confidence, 4: confident and 5: very confident, the average of scores of 1, 2, 4 and 5 could not so precisely be said to be 3 (uncertain of level of confidence). There is also not the same certainty of what these terms mean as there is for the measurement of mcg and not necessarily an equal difference in distance between 'uncertain' and 'not at all confident' as there is between 'uncertain' and 'very confident'. For ordinal data, usually the mode or median are the more appropriate descriptive statistics, although there is debate over this. For example, while their use in this situation is controversial, mean scores are often seen in the reporting of findings from Likert-type scales (Blaikie, 2003; Jamieson 2002). For nominal data the mode is usually the most appropriate. Percentage values can also be used as a descriptive statistic, but they do not tell you the central tendency.

Descriptive statistics give you a general idea of the findings from a sample, but they do not indicate how likely they are to apply to a whole population. Some studies do not have enough participants or the right sampling scheme to go beyond using descriptive statistics, and some only aim to provide a description, so they do not need to use anything else. That does not mean that the findings should not be used, but they should probably be used with caution. Jo may find an assessment tool which is reported to work well in assessing young people's emotional needs, but which has been trialled on a small sample with the data analysed using descriptive statistics. She could probably use it, but with caution, because she will not know how likely these findings are to apply to the entire population of young people.

Because mean, median, mode or percentage values do not show the spread of scores across a study group, you do not know what range of responses there were. If Jo reads a report on how long it took nurses to complete an assessment, a mean score of 36 minutes tells her than on average it took 36 minutes for it to be completed, but that does not tell her whether more or less everyone took about this time or whether it took some people an hour and some people 10 minutes. It is therefore often useful to look at how much spread there is around the mean score. This can be achieved using measures of dispersion such as the Standard Deviation (for parametric data) that show how much variation there is from the average (Thomas, 2004). A low standard deviation (SD) means that all the data are clustered close to the mean, for example, a low standard deviation might be 30–42 minutes, whereas a high-standard deviation might be between 10 minutes and 1 hour.

Inferential statistics

If Jo finds a study about an assessment tool for young people which claims that the tool is very effective, it will be useful for her to know how confident she can be that the findings will apply to any young person who is admitted to her unit. Inferential statistics are designed to give an indication of this, by suggesting how generalizable the findings are. The type of data which have been gathered again dictates whether parametric or non-parametric tests should be used. Having chosen the right menu (parametric or non-parametric), which specific test is appropriate then depends on what is being studied, for example, whether comparisons are being made, and if so, how many. There are a whole range of statistical tests which can be used, and unless your main interest in life is stats (in which case I hope you skipped this chapter), you do not really need to know them all and how they all work. If they are used in a study which you read, you can look them up and check whether they were right for what was being done. A possible flowchart for such decisions, including some of the most commonly used tests, is seen in Appendix 2.

Some of the most commonly used tests in inferential statistics are

Parametric tests
T-Test: This compares the results from two groups. It can be a one-sample t-test which compares the mean of a single group against a hypothetical or 'expected' mean or a two sample t test which compares the means of two 'real' groups.

Analysis of Variance (ANOVA): ANOVA is used to compare the means of more than two groups. A one way ANOVA is used to compare the data one way. For example, a control group compared with two different intervention groups. A two way ANOVA is used when the intention is to compare two or more groups but also compare more than one characteristic within the groups. For example, in a study with three different interventions ANOVA could be used to compare the groups as a whole, but also to compare the findings between males and females.

Non-parametric tests
Chi-Square: Chi-square is used to compare observed data with the data you would expect to obtain according to a specific hypothesis. If you toss a coin 20 times, you might expect to get ten heads and ten tails. If you got eight heads and 12 tails you could do a chi-square test to assess whether this was likely to be due to chance, or other factors.

Another variation of the chi-square test, the chi-square test for independence, can be used to determine the relationship between two variables. A study which Jo reads about medical and nursing staffs' views on a new assessment tool might look at the variable of whether nursing staff or medical staff were more enthusiastic about its use. To test whether enthusiasm for the tool is independent of (or related to) being in one of those two professional groups, the chi-square test of independence could be used.

Wilcoxon's Test and the Mann-Whitney U Test: These test for differences between two groups but use median rather than mean values (a non-parametric version of a t-test).

Kruskal-Wallis: This tests for differences between the median scores of more than two groups (a nonparametric ANOVA).

Correlation and regression
These tests are used to see whether variables are related to each other. Correlation analysis shows the direction and strength any relationship between two variables using values from -1.00 (a perfect negative correlation: as one variable increases in size, the other decreases) to 1.00 (a perfect positive correlation: as one variable increases so does the other). When the value is 0.00 there is no relationship between the two variables (Hill and Lewicki, 2007). If the correlation analysis shows that there is a relationship of some kind between variables, it is possible to try to make a prediction for one variable based on the value of another. This is done using regression analysis. Pearson's r is one of the commonly used parametric correlation and regression tests. Spearman's correlation is a non-parametric correlation test.

Tails on tests
The term 'tail' refers to the extreme of something. Tails in statistics refer to the extremes or outer edges of the curves on graphs, and a test that has 'tails' separately analyses the data which would be at the ends of the curves on a graph if the data was presented that way (Greenhalgh, 2010). A one-tailed test analyses the information at one extreme of the graph and a two-tailed test analyses the information at both ends. It means that you can see whether the people who did not fall very close to the middle or most frequent point of the graph were any different from the rest.

In the reporting of these statistical tests, a range of letters and values appear depending on the test used, but one which is consistently important is the p value. The Power is also relevant.

The p value and Power

The specific test which is performed (such as t-test, chi-square etc) analyses the data itself, and a p value is then calculated to tell you whether these results are likely to be due to chance, rather than the intervention or procedure (Thomas, 2005). Usually for something to be significant (or fairly safely generalizable) the calculated p value needs to be less than 0.05 (Thomas, 2005). The power, if commented on, should be more than 0.80. If you want more details, read on.

Two types of error can be made when a hypothesis is tested: type I and type II errors (Windish and Diener-West, 2006):

Type-I error: p value
A type I error means rejecting the null hypothesis when it is really quite likely to be true (saying something makes a difference when it is very unlikely that it does) (Windish and Diener-West, 2006). A study may have the null hypothesis

that a new assessment tool makes no difference to how young people's needs are managed. If this was erroneously rejected, it would suggest that the assessment tool does make a difference, when in fact there is no evidence that this is so. The risk of this type of error having been made is dealt with using p values.

The p value in a study refers to the chance of the null hypothesis being correct. A p value of 0.05 means that there is a 5 per cent chance that the null hypothesis is correct (or should be upheld). Conversely, there is a 95 per cent chance that it is wrong (or should not be upheld). So, by association, there is a 95 per cent chance that the hypothesis is upheld. A p value of 0.05 means that you can be 95 per cent sure that the hypothesis is upheld and that the apparent findings are not just due to chance. If the null hypothesis is that an assessment tool made no difference, and the p value for the statistical test used was reported as 0.05, then you would be able to be 95 per cent certain that the tool did make a difference and that the difference seen was due to the tool, not chance.

The level at which findings are significant enough to be generalized is usually set at 0.05 because 95 per cent certainty is generally accepted to be a reasonable level of risk. The lower the p value, the less likely it is that the null hypothesis is true (e.g., $p = 0.04$ means there is a 4 per cent chance that the null hypothesis is true and a 96 per cent chance that it is not: a 96 per cent chance that the hypothesis is upheld). So, the lower the p value, the more 'statistically significant' the result is in showing that the hypothesis is upheld, and the more confidently you can use the findings.

Type II error: power
This is about failing to reject a null hypothesis when it is false (Windish and Diener-West, 2006). If the null hypothesis of a study is that an assessment tool makes no difference, failing to reject it means that you claim that the tool makes no difference and thus recommend that it should not be used. A type II error would occur if the evidence is in fact that an assessment tool may make a difference, and there might be value in using it. The risk of this type of error is dealt with using power calculations. As the power of a test increases, the chances of making a Type II error decrease. Power analysis can be used before carrying out a study to calculate the minimum sample size required to reduce the chances of erroneously upholding the null hypothesis and by inference erroneously rejecting the hypothesis to a minimum. It can also be used once data have been collected to calculate the likelihood of the null hypothesis having been falsely accepted. Although there are no formal standards for power, most researchers accept 0.80 as a reasonable level of certainty. If the power calculation comes out as less than this, the chances of having made a type II error are higher than is usually considered acceptable (Hill and Lewicki, 2007).

So, in summary, p value and power are different calculations that tell you the chances of the study having got the wrong answer or got the answer they got just by chance, not because of anything that was actually happening in the study.

Confidence interval

A study's confidence interval (CI) tells you how precise the result is. A study might show that from a survey of 100 staff the mean time taken to complete a new assessment form was 28 minutes. The confidence interval and score tells you how precisely this probably reflects the experience of the whole population of staff working in this area. That is, the range within which one can be confident that the true result from a population rather than just the sample tested will lie (Thomas, 2005). The confidence interval might be 20–40, meaning that there is a degree of confidence that while not everyone would take 28 minutes to complete the form, most people will take between 20–40 minutes. The end points of the confidence interval are referred to as confidence limits (20–40 in this case). The confidence interval is qualified by a level of confidence, usually expressed as a percentage, about how confident the researcher is that this interval will apply to the general population. 95 per cent certainty is generally considered high enough for researchers to draw conclusions that can be generalized from samples to populations (Thomas, 2005). If a study reported that a survey of 1000 staff showed that the mean time taken to complete an assessment was 28 minutes, the confidence interval was 20–40 and the level of confidence 95 per cent, it would mean that the researcher was 95 per cent confident that all staff in the general population would take between 20–40 minutes to complete the assessment (Windish and Diener-West, 2006). This would be described as the 95 per cent confidence interval being 20–40 minutes.

The tests and scores listed above are a guide to what is seen as usually acceptable, and if what you are told is different you should question why: especially if no explanation is given. You should also consider what the tests and scores mean in terms of practical application, for instance, how vital high level generalizability is. If a study tested how well parachutes open when one hops out of a plane mid-flight, I probably would not want to voluntarily jump out of the plane unless it was about to crash with a p value of more than 0.05. A less than 95 per cent chance that the parachute will open seems unattractive. I would probably be looking for a p value somewhere close to 0.001, or lower if possible. However, if the research was about what the most cost-effective mobile phone was, I might accept descriptive statistics if they were done well, or inferential statistics with a significance of p = 0.08 because it is less likely that I would die if it turned out that the findings were not really so generalizable after all.

Results

The results from quantitative research are largely linked with the statistical tests used, and when you read the results the main things to look at are

- Were appropriate tests done for the sample size, type and distribution of data?
- Were the right tests done for what the research was looking at?

- If the study said it was comparing two (or more) things, do the results show that comparison?
- Were there any missing results? If so, would they be important? Sometimes results are missing because the study was huge and a 5000-word paper is not enough to report it all, so the authors have sensibly decided to report a meaningful chunk, and reported other bits in other papers. The time when missing data or statistics are important is if it looks as if they are being missed out so as to give a false impression. If a study was about how effective a tool was in assessing the needs of young people aged 12–18 but there were no data for the 12–14 age group and no reason given for this, Jo would want to know why.
- Do the results that the study says are significant seem to be significant? For example, does the p value listed as significant look significant. If not, is a reason given for this?

It is also important to see if there is any evidence that the researchers thought about other possible explanations for the results, for example, any confounding variables (things that could be the real reason for the study outcomes rather than the given reason).

Conclusions and recommendations

The conclusions and recommendations from a study should fit the rest of the study, and in particular the results. For example, if the results are statistically insignificant, or if there are possible confounding variables, the conclusions and recommendations should be suitably cautious. It is important to check whether anything in the conclusions seems to be overstated in light of the study design and findings. Equally though, whether anything is understated or any important links missed or not reported on matters.

Application to practice

Quantitative research is useful in practice situations where you want to know with some degree of certainty whether something will work or not and whether it can be applied with reasonable confidence of success to anyone in a given group. What it cannot tell you is the individual factors which may influence whether something will work or not, or be something which someone values or not. Jo may find a study which shows beyond reasonable doubt that a certain assessment tool will very accurately assess a young person's mental health needs. What it may not tell her is whether staff will be prepared to use it, because it will not tell her the attitudes, values and priorities which may influence this. It also cannot tell her whether it will positively influence care because that depends on what is done with the assessment. However, it may tell her whether, all things being equal, if the tool is used properly, it will provide an accurate assessment.

Summary

Quantitative research uses numbers to assess things and present information, often with the intention of showing how likely it is that the findings which have been generated can be confidently applied to whole populations. There are a range of study designs and methodologies which can be used, and a number of methods which can be employed to gather quantitative data: the quality of the study depends on the right one being used for the right thing. Similarly, the way in which the data are analysed should be appropriate for the study design. There are numerous statistical tests which can be employed to interpret quantitative data, and the right one has to be used for the right data type and study purpose. The claims to generalizability that are made should be commensurate with level of confidence which the study design, data collection and analysis processes have made possible. Like all forms of research, the key issues are whether the study was conducted systematically, and rigorously, and whether anything which could have altered what seem to be the study findings have been accounted for.

Worked examples

Sarah works in a rehabilitation service for people who have spinal injuries. The unit has ten inpatient beds, but also provides regional outpatient services. There has been a suggestion that a joint Nurse Specialist, Physiotherapy and Occupational Therapy clinic should be developed, primarily to increase attendance at appointments, but also to aid in multidisciplinary communication. It seems like a good idea, but Sarah wants to find evidence on whether this approach is likely to work. She has found a number of articles on the subject, two of which are

Paper 1

Title: Joint physiotherapy and occupational therapy clinics improve attendance at outpatient services.

Hypothesis: The study hypothesis is that holding joint physiotherapy and occupational therapy clinics increases attendance at outpatient services. The null hypothesis is that holding joint physiotherapy and occupational therapy clinics do not alter attendance at outpatient services.

Methodology and methods: The study is described as a randomized controlled trial. It was carried out at a large university hospital in a city in the UK. Non-attendance rates were recorded for physiotherapy only, occupational therapy only and the joint clinic over a one year period.

Sample: The sample was 244 adults who were referred to physiotherapy and occupational therapy services from a rheumatology department. They were randomly allocated to attend standard (separate) clinics or a joint clinic. The inclusion criteria were those who had both physiotherapy and occupational therapy appointments at the time of entering the study and the exclusion criteria those who had only a physiotherapy or occupational therapy appointment at the time of entering the study.

Ethical issues: The study was approved by an NHS research ethics committee.

Data analysis: Comparisons were made between attendance at occupational therapy only clinics and joint clinics and between physiotherapy only and joint clinics. Data were initially compared using percentage values: comparing the percentage of attendance and non attendance at the clinic types. This was described as being 'followed by' using a chi-square test to analyse the statistical significance of the scores.

Results: The analysis using percentage values showed that non-attendance at occupational therapy clinics was higher than at joint clinics (8.2% non-attendance at joint clinics compared to 19.6% non-attendance at single clinics) When analysed using chi square test the level of significance of this difference was $p = 0.01$. Non-attendance at physiotherapy clinics was also higher than at joint clinics, with an 8.2% non-attendance at joint clinics compared to 16.3% at single clinics. When analysed using chi-square test, the level of significance of this difference was $p = 0.05$. These differences were therefore statistically significant and the hypothesis was upheld. The data were not analysed against any variable such as sex and age.

Conclusion: The conclusion was that joint appointments appear to improve attendance at outpatients appointments.

Evaluation

Hypotheses: The hypothesis suggests that this paper may be useful. There is a hypothesis and corresponding null hypothesis.

Methodology: The study used quantitative methodology, which is appropriate for gathering numerical data from which there is an intention to generalize, as was the case in this study.

Study design: This was an experimental study, and an RCT is the Gold Standard way of conducting an experiment. The comparison between an experimental (joint appointment) and control (separate OT and physiotherapy appointments) group should make meaningful comparisons possible. Randomization was used, which reduces the risk of any apparent findings being due to chance or bias from the patients placed in each group. It would not have been possible to blind in this study, because patients and therapists would have known which group they were in. The study seemed to measure what it was intended to: that is, attendance or non-attendance at clinics. It considered the potentially confounding variable of physiotherapy versus occupational therapy clinic rather than solely joint versus single clinics. However the potential variables of sex and age were not compared. Diagnosis was not considered, but this might have been impossible and the broad remit of rheumatology is probably sufficient.

Sample: Randomization would have reduced bias, as there was an equal chance of each individual being in either group. There was no suggestion that a power calculation was used to determine the ideal sample size.

Ethical issues: Ethics approval was granted. Whether patients consented to participate was not clear, but with ethical clearance this could probably be assumed to be the case.

Analysis: The data were non-parametric ('attend' and 'did not attend', with no numerical values). Descriptive statistics (percentage values) were initially used which gave an overall impression of the findings, but did not address generalizability. Chi-square was a suitable inferential test, as it is non-parametric and will test whether or not in this case attendance at outpatients was independent of the type of clinic. Technically it is not correct to say that the chi-square test 'followed on' from the percentage scores, because percentage scores do not show the central tendency. However, using both ways of analysing data were appropriate for their specific purposes.

Results: There was a numerical difference in attendance figures, and this was shown to be statistically significant ($p = 0.01$ and 0.05) meaning that there is a 99% and 95% chance respectively that any differences detected in attendance at the joint rather than single speciality clinic was due to the clinic types being used, not chance.

Conclusions: These fit the results, and the hypothesis was upheld. It would be worth Sarah taking these findings into account along with the other evidence she gathers. The study did not include a tripartite approach (Occupational Therapy, Physiotherapy and Clinical nurse specialist) so it is not directly transferable to Sarah's situation, but may be a useful source of information.

The study only dealt with non-attendance: multidisciplinary communication, which also interests Sarah, was not discussed.

Paper 2

Title: Does using a shared clinic improve attendance at outpatients appointments?

Aims: The aim of the study was to determine whether attendance at medical neurology outpatients appointments was increased by patients seeing an occupational therapist and/or physiotherapist and physician at the same clinic.

Methodology: The study was a comparative study. The comparison was between the new appointment system (seeing a neurologist and one or more other professionals at one clinic), or only seeing a physician. The measure of interest was non-attendance.

Methods: The study was conducted one year after the introduction of a new one appointment clinic system. It measured the number of failures to attend (DNA) neurology outpatients appointments in the year following the introduction of the new system (prospective data) compared with the DNAs in the previous year (retrospective data).

Sample: The total number of patients who were sent appointments in the retrospective sample was 1010 compared to 1072 in the prospective part of the study. The criteria were that to be included in the study patients had to require physiotherapy and/or occupational therapy appointments as well as neurology appointments.

Ethical issues: The study was approved by the NHS Research Ethics Committee.

Data analysis: A chi-square test was used

Results: There were fewer DNAs in the year following the introduction of the new appointments system ($p = 0.04$) (fewer DNAs when patients were seen by a neurologist and another professional).

Conclusions: The conclusion was that joint clinics increase attendance at neurology outpatients appointments.

Evaluation

Research question: This study's title seems relevant, but it does not investigate exactly what Sarah is interested in.

Methodology: Quantitative methods are an appropriate approach for this type of comparison which seeks to numerically evaluate the effect of a change in service provision.

Research design: This is a comparative study, comparing two things: attendance at a clinic where only the physician is seen to one where a physician and another professional are seen. It is not a case-control study, cross sectional study or longitudinal study: it is a simple comparison using prospective and retrospective data. This is probably a sensible approach because only this type of data were available if a concurrent trial was not achievable. However, the reliability of data might be affected by any changes in the department in question which could have influenced attendance other than the new method of providing clinics. The measurement seems valid, because it measures non-attendance, which is the focus of the paper.

Sample: The sample was the complete population of those invited to appointments in the years in question and who met the inclusion criteria. It was a large sample although no evidence was provided of a power calculation being undertaken before the study. The groups were not matched numerically, because they were the total number of attendees over a year. While randomization and controlling were not possible, the study design did not claim this. The variables of age and sex, any whether the patients attended appointments where they saw a physician, occupational therapist and physiotherapist; physician and occupational therapist; or physician and physiotherapist were not considered. The comparison was only between joint clinics and medic only clinics.

Analysis: The data gathered was non-parametric ('yes' 'no' to attendance, nominal data). Chi-square is an appropriate statistical test for comparing 2 sets of non parametric data. As nominal data were used, a Wilcoxon's Test or Mann-Whitney U Test which test for differences between two groups but use median values would be problematic.

Results: The results suggest that the joint clinic approach significantly improved appointment attendance ($p = 0.04$: suggests a 96% chance that the null hypothesis should be rejected and only 4% chance that it would be falsely rejected: a 96% chance that improved attendance was due to the joint clinic, not chance).

Conclusions: These fit the results as presented but again the primary outcome was attendance, not communication.

This study appears to show significant results from a reasonably well designed study, however it does not exactly match what Sarah is interested in, as the focus was on increasing attendance at physicians' appointments by adding in occupational therapy and/or physiotherapy appointments. Whether attendance at physiotherapy and occupational therapy appointments was improved by this mechanism was not considered. Only attendance was noted, not any aspects of interprofessional communication which Sarah is also interested in.

Taken together, these two papers, while very different, suggest that the idea of joint clinics merits further exploration.

Appraising qualitative research

6

Scenario

Anthony has just taken a job in the community, working with people with severe learning disabilities. A significant part of his job is working with the families who provide for the day-to-day care needs of his client group. He is looking for research which will help him to better understand the needs of these families, and thinks that he might be better off looking at qualitative rather than quantitative enquiry.

Principles of qualitative enquiry

Qualitative research does not aim to produce findings which are generalizable to an entire population, instead, it explores issues that are likely to be subjective and very individual (Davies *et al.*, 2009; Polkinghorne, 2005). It would be inappropriate to say that a qualitative study was flawed because it was not generalizable. It is not meant to be. Anthony is right to think that qualitative enquiry may help him to understand the needs of the families of people who have severe learning disabilities. The information will not be the type which he can guarantee will apply to every family he works with, but it will be useful to enable him to gain insight into people's experiences, and the numerous and subjective factors which can impact on these.

Situations in which qualitative enquiry may be useful

The intention of qualitative research is not to provide a solution which can be applied in all situations. It generally aims to provide an in-depth exploration of individuals' experiences of a particular situation (for example, having a child who has severe learning disabilities), in order to improve our understanding of how people might experience, view or understand that situation (Lo Bindo-Wood and Haber, 2005). Anthony may find a qualitative study which shows the problems which a particular family experienced when trying to organize their child's post-compulsory education. This could include the difficulties they encountered when services did not work together, a lack of post-compulsory education opportunities for this client group and perhaps issues to do with transport. However, these findings would not mean that all families will experience these problems, or experience them in the same way. What it means is that Anthony will be aware that these issues may exist, and be better placed to work proactively with families, but hopefully without being a prophet of unnecessary doom for those who do not have any problems in this respect.

Research question

Because qualitative research does not aim to show anything beyond reasonable doubt, generalize findings to an entire population or use statistical analysis, there is no hypothesis (Ryan, Coughlan and Cronin, 2007). However, the purpose of the study should be clear. One additional consideration in qualitative research is that some approaches allow for the research question or focus to be modified as new data develop understanding about what is being studied (Ryan, Coughlan and Cronin, 2007). If the conclusions seem to be about something slightly different from where the research started, that may be acceptable, as long as the rationale for this is given, and seems reasonable. A study which started out looking at education provision for young adults with severe learning difficulties might end up focusing on transport if the initial data-collection activities identified this as a major issue. That would be quite acceptable, provided that how and why this decision was made clear in the study report.

Literature review

The literature review in a research report should usually provide an objective account of the existing evidence on a subject, to demonstrate why the study was carried out and how it contributes to the existing knowledge base (Ryan, Coughlan and Cronin, 2007). Sometimes this is exactly what it does, but the literature is occasionally dealt with differently in qualitative enquiry. For example, in many types of grounded theory, data are collected in isolation from any predetermined theory. The literature review is carried out after the data have been collected, and the theory which has been generated from the data is then compared to existing literature rather than existing theory being used to inform data collection (Burns and Grove, 2005). This means that the literature review may precede or succeed data collection in qualitative research, depending on the methodology. A grounded theory study about the provision of support for families whose child has severe learning disabilities might start with discussions with families, and the theory generated from this then can be compared with the existing literature. In contrast, an ethnography on the same subject might start with a literature review. Both approaches are entirely acceptable, provided there is a good reason for it.

Methodology

There are a range of specific methodologies or approaches to qualitative research (Polkinghorne, 2005; Ponterotto, 2005), but the most commonly described are phenomenology, ethnography, grounded theory and narrative research. Although these are all qualitative methodologies, they are each influenced by different theoretical perspectives, and each methodology itself contains subdivisions of exactly how and why things are done (Russell and Gregory, 2003). However, their main principles are

Phenomenology aims to describe people's lived experiences in relation to what is being studied: their experiences of the phenomenon (Balls, 2009; Willig, 2008). Anthony might find a phenomenological study that explores parents' experiences of caring for a grown-up child who has severe learning difficulties. Phenomenology is often divided into descriptive phenomenology and interpretative (hermeneutic) phenomenology. One of the practical distinctions between these approaches is that descriptive phenomenology considers it important for the researcher to completely put aside what they already know or think about the phenomenon under investigation (a process described as bracketing) before starting to collect data, so as to approach the study with no preconceptions (Dowling, 2004; Lopez and Willis, 2004; Todres, 2005; Willig, 2008: 55–6). Interpretative phenomenology believes it is impossible to rid oneself of such preconceptions and approach a study in a completely neutral way. It acknowledges the effect which our own experiences have on how we interpret those of others, and as such these also become a part of the research data (Willig, 2008: 56–68).

Ethnography aims to provide in-depth descriptions of everyday life for individuals, groups or cultures and to explain how these create meaning for those involved (Ryan, Coughlan and Cronin, 2007). The researcher's understanding is developed through long-term engagement with the culture that is being studied, usually by extensive participant observation (Lee, 2006b). The duration of the researcher's engagement with the situation being studied (often called 'the field') depends on exactly what is being studied and in what setting. Although participant observation is the mainstay of ethnography, additional data sources, such as interviews and document analysis, are often also used (Ryan, Coughlan and Cronin, 2007). A paper which would interest Anthony might involve an ethnographer spending long periods of time with a family whose child has severe learning disabilities. This might include them observing their lives, the challenges and rewards which they face and how they manage these. Observation might be interspersed with discussion or informal interviews with family members to gain further insight into their perceptions of what is happening. The researcher might also read any diary, blog or other documents which the family allow them to, so as to broaden and deepen their insight into the family's experiences.

Grounded theory aims to develop theory about something, with the theory which is developed grounded in the data generated for the research, rather than any preconceived ideas about what that theory might be (Lee, 2006b, Ryan, Coughlan and Cronin, 2007). As the researcher begins to gather data, they develop theoretical concepts about what they are researching and, having developed these, go on to further test them in new data gathering activities (Ryan, Coughlan and Cronin, 2007). Anthony might find a grounded theory study which begins by interviewing five parents of children who have severe learning disabilities, in order to develop a theory about what service provision they need. When the researcher has developed some ideas or theories about this, they might go on to test these theories by carrying out more interviews with the same or other families to see if the ideas they have ring true or can be further developed.

Narrative research, as the name suggests, focuses on gathering narratives (which might be termed stories or accounts) from participants. The accounts are then interpreted and analysed by the researcher and presented in a way which shows context, sequence and interpretations so that each event can be seen in relation to a whole experience (Elliot, 2005). A narrative in which a researcher gathered families' stories or narratives about their lives with their children who have severe learning disabilities would arrange these into a coherent and logically proceeding whole. This would clearly identify the context in which the families' stories exist, draw out what the main issues were and how these affect and were affected by other issues.

There are also methodologies which do not conform to any one methodological model, or which combine ideas from more than one approach or philosophy. However, a commonality between all qualitative methodologies is that they gather non-numerical data, in sufficient depth to really understand all the intricacies of what is being explored.

Methods

There is no one right way to gather qualitative data: the best method is one which means that data were collected in a way that addressed the research issue, was consistent with the methodology and was likely to gain the required information (Astin 2009; Carter and Little, 2007; Lee, 2006b; Russell and Gregory, 2003).

Commonly used methods in qualitative research are interviews and observation. However open-ended questionnaires, analysis of documents (such as emails or diaries) (Brown and Lloyd, 2001) and a whole range of other methods can be used. The question to ask when reading a report is: would this method have enabled the researcher to gather data which would address the focus of the research?

Interviews are a very commonly used method in qualitative research, and are usually either semi-structured or unstructured (Lee, 2006b). Structured interviews use closed questions with yes/ no or numerical answers and are seldom appropriate for qualitative research, because they do not allow any depth of exploration of the matter in question (Whiting, 2008). Semi-structured interviews have a structure and key questions, but allow for other questions to be added and developed as the dialogue progresses. Unstructured interviews are more like conversations in which the interviewer elicits information around a set of issues but with no particular sequence or format for the questions (Whiting, 2008). These latter two approaches are the most useful in qualitative enquiry, because they allow the researcher to explore whatever is most relevant and important for the person they are interviewing, and to follow additional and unexpected leads if they arise (Burck, 2005).

Interviews may be conducted by different means: face to face, online or by telephone, with individuals or groups, as one-off interactions or a series of interviews: whatever is most likely to elicit the type of data required, and be manageable. A balance often has to be sought between the ideal and the doable: it might be ideal to carry out face-to-face interviews, but on a limited budget and with a geographically diverse group, telephone interviews might be the only feasible option. This does not invalidate the study, but it might detract from the depth of data if the participants are not as confident in chatting on the phone as they would be face to face, and because the researcher will not be able to note any non-verbal clues. Alternatively, it might make the encounter more productive because the participant may feel more comfortable talking on the telephone. Both methods have advantages and disadvantages, so it is the researcher's job to choose the one which is the most advantageous or least disadvantageous, and is doable.

Observation is also commonly used in qualitative research, and involves the researcher 'getting to know' the people they are studying and their world. It ranges in approach from participant to non-participant observation (Brown and Lloyd, 2001). In participant observation, the observer seeks to experience the situation which they are studying as if they were a part of it, while also aiming to stand back a little to try to understand, analyse and explain it. Non-participant observation is where the researcher is present but does not participate in the situation being studied. However, observation does not necessarily rest on either of these extremes: it exists on a continuum in which researchers make decisions about the exact level of participation and observation that is best for the study in question. It is also possible for researchers to adopt the role of participant observer in some aspects of a study and non-participant observer in others. The role which the researcher adopted at any given point, and why this was the most suitable for the occasion and subject studied should be clear in the study report though. There should also be some evidence of the researcher considering the effect that their role might have had on the behaviour and activities of those around them (for example, changed behaviour because of participants knowing they were being observed).

Questionnaires can be designed to gather qualitative data if they use open-ended questions, and their wording encourages participants to give in-depth responses (Lee, 2006b). It can be difficult to gather truly 'qualitative' data by solely using questionnaires, because many respondents do not give extensive responses even when invited to. However, if they really do generate qualitative data, not just very short and superficial answers, they can be very useful.

Document analysis may also be used to enhance understanding of what experiences mean for individuals, groups or communities (Brown and Lloyd, 2001). This may include looking at media reports (for example, a family may have given a report to a newspaper), minutes of meetings, diaries or letters. Documents may be useful as a main data source, or in building up a fuller picture of a situation that is being primarily studied by other means. For example, an ethnography of a family whose child has severe learning disabilities might predominantly use participant observation, accompanied by some formal discussions or interviews, and analysis of a diary or blog. The aim is to build a picture of their many and varied experiences using as many sources as will usefully contribute to understanding their world.

Reflection is a key aspect of qualitative research. Qualitative enquiry is carried out in a real-life context and a part of this is acknowledging that we all have opinions, beliefs and experiences which will almost inevitably affect how we interpret, deal with and make decisions about most things in life, including research. Descriptive phenomenology requires the researcher's own existing views, values and opinions to be analysed and placed to one side before the study begins (Dowling, 2004; Lopez and Willis, 2004; Willig, 2008: 56–68), while other approaches recommend that the researcher deals with this in an ongoing manner (Willig, 2008: 56–68). What matters when you are evaluating a qualitative research report is that the researcher in some way acknowledges that their own views and experiences might impact on how data were gathered, analysed or interpreted and explains the steps they took to address this. This may include making notes that discuss how their input into interviews, conversation etc. might have affected the responses (Whiting, 2008), or how they felt at specific points in the research, so that they can see how their analysis of the situation might have been affected by this (Burck, 2005; Hand, 2003). Their notes might also include practical challenges, tiredness, anything which might affect the research process and decision-making trail. This is often achieved by the researcher keeping a field journal or diary which they use in the analysis and interpretation of data.

Triangulation of data is often referred to: this means using more than one method of gathering data to create a more complete picture of the subject under investigation (McBrien, 2008). Data sources which are triangulated might be observation and interviews; document analysis, observation and questionnaires or any other combination. The intention is not necessarily to see if the data sources agree with each other, but to use them as different angles to gain a fuller impression of the matter being researched, including contradictions, and views which seem contextual and changeable (McBrien, 2008).

Sampling

Sample sizes in qualitative research are often small (Fossey *et al.*, 2002) but because the aim is not to generalize the findings, this is not a problem. Studies which have too many participants can in fact be problematic, because a large sample may mean that the depth of enquiry required has not been achieved. The concern in qualitative enquiry is not how many people were involved, but whether data were collected in sufficient depth to bring about understanding (Polkinghorne, 2005).

The end point of data collection in qualitative research is often not prespecified because this depends on the data which are gathered. Data collection usually stops when the researcher feels that the data they have provides enough depth of information. This occurs when the researcher notes that no new insights or leads are being offered, and no new theory being generated: a point referred to as data saturation (Bradley, Curry and Devers, 2007; Parahoo, 2006). However, Thorne and Darbyshire (2005) suggest that some researchers use the term 'data saturation' as meaning a convenient stopping point for their study rather than really achieving saturation. It may be pertinent to try to assess whether a study seems likely to have achieved true data saturation, for example, from the number and duration of interviews carried out, or the length of time spent in the field of enquiry as well as whether the researcher used this term. However, even if a study has not achieved data saturation, the findings may still be useful. The decision related to using research in practice is not so much whether, strictly speaking, data saturation was achieved, but whether the insights offered are sufficiently rich and contextualized to be of use.

Purposive sampling is often used in qualitative enquiry (Ryan, Coughlan and Cronin, 2007). Because the aim of qualitative research is to ensure richness and depth of exploration, not representativeness of the population as a whole (Fossey *et al.*, 2002; Polkinghorne, 2005), the participants often have to be specifically, or purposefully, sought out. In some cases, further selection criteria are decided on and additional participants recruited (often using snowballing sampling) during data collection (Polkinghorne, 2005). In grounded theory studies, as the researcher begins to develop a theory, they may need to seek out more participants with specific experiences who are likely to be able to contribute to the development of this theory. Anthony might find a study in which the researcher interviewed six parents whose children had severe learning disabilities. If the participants highlighted the problem of getting on well with the staff who provide their day-to-day support, and one of them mentioned a friend who had decided to use a Personal Budget for her child in an attempt to overcome this problem, the researcher could usefully ask if they could speak with that person. They would be an important data source because of their experience of a specific and important way of approaching care provision, and thus it would be perfectly legitimate to seek them out. It would, in this type of enquiry, probably be remiss not to at least try to contact and see if they would be prepared to participate in the study. As well as it not being necessary to prespecify the sample in this type of research, this may be deleterious to the enquiry if it means that important data are overlooked.

Data analysis

Qualitative data analysis almost always involves the transformation of vast quantities of data into a coherent set of categories, a description, narrative or theory which very clearly addresses the research question, issue or problem. Exactly how this is achieved depends on the methodology and methods used (Vishnevsky and Beanlands, 2004). However, the focus is usually on analysing text and presenting this as words, meanings and interpretations, not numbers.

Analysis of qualitative data can include both the precise words recorded and transcribed, and the interpretation which the researcher gives to these (Campos and Turato, 2009). Data are usually initially organized by using a set of codes that are applied to sections of data which seem to have a particular meaning. These coded sections are then arranged into themes or categories: collections of coded sections which have a common thread (Balls, 2009; Burla *et al.*, 2008; Campos and Turato, 2009). Exactly how this is achieved varies, but the process of breaking volumes of data into meaningful chunks and then piecing these back together, with those deemed to have similar meanings together, in order to understand the whole, is the essence of qualitative analysis and interpretation (Campos and Turato, 2009).

The codes which are used to describe data chunks may be developed inductively or deductively, or by using a combination of induction and deduction depending on the nature and aims of the study (Bradley, Curry and Devers, 2007). In deductive coding, topics of interest or codes are chosen before the data are analysed. The opposite is true in inductive coding: codes are developed by reading through the data and seeing what ideas are generated from it. These ideas become, or strongly direct, the codes (Bradley, Curry and Devers, 2007).

Some ways of analysing qualitative data require that only one code is used per section of data, and stipulate that codes cannot be placed into more than one category. However in many cases, segments of data can and indeed should be allocated more than one code because the intertwined nature of human experiences often makes mutually exclusive categories impossible (Graneheim and Lundman, 2004). For example, if the mother of a young man who had severe learning disabilities described her experience of organizing a holiday by saying

It took three months to organize. The cost, a place that could cater for his needs, organizing transport and care staff. It was exhausting, but it also made me angry, because it's just so hard to organize these things, it would be important for this paragraph to be seen in the context of other data coded as 'holidays', 'cost', 'provision by society', 'anger', 'exhaustion' 'staffing' and 'transport'. Limiting this paragraph to one code might mean that some areas of data analysis were missing an important piece of the jigsaw puzzle: to omit this piece of information from a code about 'cost' might mean that the additional cost which parents whose children have severe learning disabilities can face when organizing holidays was lost. However, if a paper reports that its principles were that only one code was used for each section, this is acceptable, as long as the rationale is clear and this fits the overall study design and ethos.

There is also a discussion about whether one or more person carrying out the coding in a qualitative study is better. Coding in large studies is often done by more than one person because, practically, it has to be, and using more than one person can reduce the effect of the researcher's subjective views on data interpretation. However, it does mean that the codes need to be very clearly defined and the rules for their application consistent, which can be a challenge, especially when new codes are being developed as the study progresses (Burla *et al.*, 2008). In approaches such as grounded theory it is not usually appropriate to use more than one coder, because the study will not operate a predefined coding system: coding develops as the study progresses, almost simultaneously with data collection (Burla *et al.*, 2008). If more than one coder is used, the level of inter coder agreement, and the level at which this will be deemed to be acceptable, must be determined. This can be achieved using methods such as Kappa where a set number of transcripts are coded independently and then compared for consistency of application of codes (Burla *et al.*, 2008). The research team has to decide whether the particular type of qualitative research is appropriate for using more than one coder, and whether this will enhance or detract from study quality (Burla *et al.*, 2008). Like most aspects of qualitative enquiry, no one thing is right for all studies. The thing to look at is what was right for the study in question.

The process of analysing the data from a qualitative study should ideally be described in sufficient detail to enable the reader to judge whether the final outcome is a true or accurate representation of the data gathered (Thorne and Darbyshire, 2005).

Truth of data

The main issue in adopting (or not) the findings from any research comes down to the question: are the findings true and the conclusions and recommendations reasonable?

There has been a great deal of discussion over how the quality or truth of qualitative research can be judged (Hoye and Severinsson, 2007; Tobin and Begley, 2004). Because the aim of qualitative research is very different from quantitative research, the same rules cannot be used to assess its worth. Instead, ways of assessing the quality of a study which match its nature need to be applied. The variety of approaches to qualitative enquiry that exist makes having one set of criteria which will be precisely applicable to them all almost impossible. However, it is often seen as necessary to have some criteria or guidelines with which to evaluate qualitative studies (Dixon-Woods *et al.*, 2004). Criteria proposed by Lincoln and Guba (1985) for evaluating what is termed a study's trustworthiness are frequently cited as being useful in this respect. These criteria are credibility, dependability, transferability and confirmability.

The trustworthiness of a study essentially deals with how much trust or confidence you should have that the findings are true. Qualitative enquiry acknowledges the subjectivity of what we see as 'truth', and trustworthiness is not about whether the research participants told the truth, but about whether the researcher has faithfully represented what they have been presented with. Anthony may read a study in which a family describes how they were refused any assistance with their child's education. It may not be entirely 'true' that this was the case. They may have had some assistance which they had forgotten about, or they may not have recognized that something was aimed at assisting them. The truth that is important for Anthony is not so much whether that family did or did not receive help, but rather that whether they believed they did, and their feelings about this, not the researcher's views of reality, were represented.

Credibility deals with the confidence one has in how far the processes of gathering and analysing data meant that the study's intended focus was addressed (Graneheim and Lundman 2004). This includes using the right methods to gather data, whether data triangulation was used, the sample and sampling methods, the context of the study, prolonged engagement, depth of interviewing, whether detailed notes were kept and how data were analysed (Roberts and Priest, 2006).

Credibility also concerns whether there is consistency between the research participants' views and the researcher's representation of these. This can be almost impossible for the reader of a research report to really know, because you will probably not know the participants, or have seen all the data that were gathered; but you can assess whether steps were taken to make sure this was likely to be the case. Credibility may be enhanced by the researcher interpreting how their own experiences, input or presence affected the research, and by them consulting with participants to check that their views have been faithfully represented (known as respondent validation or member checking) (Koch, 2006; Roberts and Priest, 2006; Russell and Gregory, 2003). Asking people to confirm your interpretation of their thoughts is always useful. We have probably all had the experience of people thinking they understood what we said, and acting on or repeating this, when that was not what we meant at all. Respondent validation aims to overcome 'That is not what I said at all!' problem in research.

The value of seeking respondent validation has, nonetheless, been debated (Graneheim and Lundman, 2004). What respondents are being asked to validate must be established: for instance, whether they are looking at the interview transcripts to make sure that the researcher heard correctly, or to confirm their interpretations and conclusions. A decision also has to be made as to what will happen if respondents disagree with how they are portrayed but the researcher believes this to be a true interpretation. In group-interview settings, it may be difficult to check interpretations with all the group members. Instead the person facilitating the discussion may stop intermittently and summarize what seem to be the main points so far, in order to confirm this with the participants. In some circumstances respondent validation may not be feasible or desirable, but it is useful to see if this was considered, and, if it was not, the reason for this.

Dependability is about whether the report gives sufficient information about the research processes and how the conclusions were reached (Koch, 2006). It links to the concept of the data gathered being auditable (auditability). This may include saying how codes were developed, and describing the thought processes involved in decision making. However, the word counts allowed in journals do not usually allow for great depth of discussion of such processes (Dickie, 2003). Thus, it may be something which, while desirable, is not easy to assess in relatively short research reports.

Transferability concerns the extent to which findings can be transferred to other situations or groups. While the intention of qualitative research is not to generalize findings, you do need to know if it is likely to apply to your area of work. This requires the report to give a detailed enough description of the setting and context of the study, and the characteristics of participants, for you to know how close it seems to the setting to which you propose to transfer the findings (Graneheim and Lundman, 2004).

Confirmability is also sometimes referred to: this is really concerned with establishing that the findings were indeed derived from the data (Tobin and Begley, 2004). Confirmability is usually established when credibility, transferability and dependability are achieved.

There is not universal agreement among qualitative researchers that the criteria suggested by Lincoln and Guba (1985) are the best way to demonstrate study quality. Researchers who do not use these criteria may state how they evaluated the quality of their study, and many equally acceptable alternative criteria exist. As a baseline guide, and to provide some ideas which you might think about when evaluating qualitative research, Lincoln and Guba's (1985) criteria may nonetheless be useful.

A criticism of qualitative research has been that we cannot really know its quality: we did not hear the interviews, see the transcripts, etc. This is true. However, it is also true of quantitative work. We seldom see the researchers taking blood, watch the statisticians doing their work or have the full list of results to check the statistics against. We take that on trust. We have to take a great deal about published research on trust, and that trust may be misplaced. This applies to all research though: not just qualitative work.

Findings

The findings from any study should be clearly related to the research issue or question. In qualitative research this is often achieved by outlining which themes or categories relate to parts of the research aim, question or objectives. Quotations are usually used to illustrate the points being made in order to indicate how the claims to a particular finding are substantiated, or to further illustrate what the researcher meant by a point. Unlike quantitative studies, there are no specific criteria (such as checking p values) to tell you if the findings are 'significant' or should be acted upon. Instead, it is necessary to decide whether the findings suggest a richly textured and comprehensive set of data without any apparent gaps (Graneheim and Lundman, 2004; Russell and Gregory, 2003). Although quotes are usually anonymized, it can be helpful if the writer has indicated which participant's quotes they are using. If 20 people were interviewed and all the quotes in a paper are from one person, despite their views being important, it might bring into question whether the researcher has really presented the variety of views and possible contradictions which you would expect to find in the real world.

Conclusions

The claims that are made in a study's conclusion should be supported by sufficient evidence from the findings. In qualitative enquiry, the conclusions are not generalizations about what should be done in every situation, but highlight what key issues and considerations the study has unearthed, their importance and context. If you get to the conclusions and wonder how on earth the researcher concluded that, given the findings, then you probably should not use the study unless you read it again and can see why.

Applying qualitative research to practice

It is not possible to take the findings from a piece of qualitative work and give it out to everyone with confidence that they will all do better for it. It may also be much harder to state with confidence that you have used qualitative research than to do so with quantitative research. If dressing A has been shown to be the best thing to use, you can usually say with some confidence whether or not you used it. However if Anthony finds a qualitative study which illustrates the value of someone taking the time to listen to parents' concerns for their child's long-term future, it is much harder to say for sure that he has applied this knowledge to his practice. He might be able to say whether he spent time with parents, but whether he really listened, and whether the parents felt listened to, is very hard to say. What he can do is consider this, take it into account, do his best to listen for as long or as short a time as a particular parent seems to want him to, and put listening to parents' long-term concerns on his priority rather than optional extra list at work. Qualitative work is not measurable: and neither is its application.

Summary

To decide whether to use a piece of qualitative research, it is not possible to look for one set of rules which will always work. Instead, you have to keep in mind the intention of qualitative research, think about whether the way in which data were collected and analysed seem reasonable for this approach and whether they address the issue in question. Applying qualitative research in practice requires consideration of whether your workplace is similar enough to the study context for the findings to be in any way transferable, what bits are likely to be relevant and what bits are not. That is always going to be a very individual matter, which you have to weigh up.

Worked examples

Natalie works in community-based child and adolescent mental health services, and is interested in developing provision for the parents of young people who have eating disorders. She has some thoughts about what might be useful, but is also reading the literature to get other ideas and directions.

The papers which she has found include the following:

Paper 1

Title: Can't eat won't eat: living with a child who has anorexia nervosa.

Study aims: The aim of the study was to gain insight into the experience of being the parent of a child who has anorexia nervosa.

Methodology: The study used a grounded theory approach.

Methods: Repeated interviews with the parents of three teenage girls who had anorexia nervosa, conducted over a one-year period. One parent was interviewed on six occasions, and the other two on five. The decision about when to cease interviewing was described as being when data saturation was achieved. The researcher kept a journal in which she made notes related to her observations during interviews, but also her own feelings, interpretations and responses to situations. She also described attempting to approach the study without preconceived ideas of the subject in question or likely findings.

Sample: Three families were involved. One father and two mothers participated. Their children were aged 14, 14 and 16. Details of the families' structures and socio-economic status were provided. The study was conducted in the USA.

Data analysis: This was described as being thematic analysis.

Ethics approval: Approval was granted by a university ethics board. Informed consent was sought from participants.

Findings: The findings were presented within the themes which were developed. These were supported by quotes from interviews. The themes were: helplessness, anger, guilt, anxiety (for the future), fear for child's future, judgement (from professionals and society), stigma and frustration.

The conclusions were that having a child who had anorexia nervosa could affect their parents at a number of interrelated levels. On an emotional level, it could create feelings of helplessness and anxiety. Having a child with anorexia created changes in their ability to fulfil their parental roles: for example, their role as nurturer and protector was lost. This could affect their emotional state and could make them feel angry, guilty and frustrated with themselves and their child. Their anger and frustration could also extend to service providers who seemed incapable of improving things. Anorexia extended its influence to the family's social events and had a stigma for the child and family which in turn affected their roles and emotional well-being.

The study stated that it offered an in-depth exploration of these families' experiences and from it developed a theory of how the aspects of having a child who had anorexia were complex and interrelated. While the intention was not to achieve generalizability, it suggested that the findings could have resonance for other families and situations.

Evaluation

Aim: This paper seems very relevant to Natalie's work.

Methodology: The subject seems appropriate for the qualitative paradigm, with grounded theory as a methodology. The intention was to gather in-depth understanding of a real-life situation, in the context in which it happened and to develop theory from this. The researcher explained how she had attempted to approach the situation without preconceptions about the subject or likely findings.

Methods: These seem appropriate for the study. Repeated interviews would allow in-depth exploration of information, and enable theory to be developed, checked and expanded in the light of what seemed to be the initial findings.

Sample: The study involved three parents, one father and two mothers. This number of participants would allow the depth of engagement required in qualitative enquiry. How the families were selected was not clear, but this is probably not important in deciding whether to use the information in the study in practice.

Ethical issues: Informed consent was gained and approval was given by a relevant ethics board.

Data analysis: Data were analysed using an appropriate approach.

Credibility is addressed by prolonged engagement, the researcher continuing to gather data until saturation was achieved, notes being kept by the researcher, including notes about their own feelings and responses in the research situation, and appropriate methods being used. Respondent validation was achieved by ongoing checking of findings and ideas in ongoing interviews. How the themes were developed is not stated, but this is possibly due to the journal article limits, so dependability/auditability is difficult to judge. The context is described which allows the reader to assess the transferability of the findings. Thus, the study seems reasonably trustworthy.

Findings and conclusions: The findings are clear and the conclusions and theory developed seem to be derived from these. This paper, while offering what may be unique insights, seems worthy of noting in developing services. That it was conducted in the USA may limit some aspects of application to the UK, for example, methods of service provision. The paper does not make specific recommendations which can be implemented, but the issues which are raised are likely to be useful in focusing Natalie's thoughts on what provision might be useful for parents.

Paper 2

Title: Parents' experiences of having a child who is anorexic.

Aim: The paper aimed to explore the experiences of parents who have a child with anorexia nervosa.

Methodology: The study used a qualitative methodology (no specific statement of methodology other than this was provided).

Methods: Focus group interviews with parents whose child has anorexia. A semi-structured interview schedule was used.
    Interviews lasted between1 hour and 90 minutes. They were taped and transcribed. The same interviewer facilitated all the groups.

Sample: A total of 22 parents were involved. The focus groups had about 5–6 participants each. Four groups were held. Although a mix of fathers and mothers were invited, of the 22 participants only four were fathers. These were split between two of the groups. The sample is described as a convenience volunteer sample generated by advertising in health centres and locations which provided care for young people with anorexia nervosa.

Ethics: NHS ethics committee approval was given. Participants were advised that their identities would remain confidential but also reminded that the group itself had a responsibility to maintain confidentiality regarding the information provided by others and group membership.

Data analysis: This was described as inductive analysis of interview transcripts using codes and developing categories to present key themes.

Findings: The findings were grouped under headings from the categories developed and the codes and categories described were supported by quotes from a range of parents. The headings were: emotional load poorly recognized, care needs poorly recognized, lack of support, blame, guilt, uncertainty and fear.

Conclusions: Parents felt that the emotional load of caring for a child with anorexia, their practical care needs and the impact on their lives were poorly recognized. The suggestion was that parents generally felt unsupported and often blamed for their child's condition, which compounded their feelings of guilt. They often felt unsure of what was expected of them and how to best help their child. They feared for their child's future, both in terms of education and employment, but also for their long term health.
    The conclusion indicated that the study had sought to understand, in some depth, the experiences of parents, and to convey individual and contextual experiences. While it did not claim to be generalizable, it suggested that the study had highlighted many issues which practitioners should consider.

Evaluation

Aim: This seems a relevant subject.

Methodology: The study uses qualitative methodology which is suitable for gaining insight into people's lived experiences. A specific type of qualitative methodology is not described, which is not a problem, provided that the decisions made within the study are consistent with each other. It is usually preferable if a study which does not exactly match one approach or methodology does not try to claim to do so.

Methods: Focus groups have pros and cons, but the rationale for using them was reasoned and reasonable. The number of participants in each group was acceptable: enough to generate a range of ideas and perspectives but not so many that inadequate depth of data were generated, large enough to generate discussion but not so large that some participants would be unable to contribute. There was no indication of whether any group members dominated or seemed less participative than others so the assumption is that the groups 'worked'. The interviews lasted between 1 hour and 90 minutes each, which suggests some depth of discussion.

Sample: The sample was a convenience sample, composed of volunteers, which means that it is likely that those who were particularly keen to share experiences or views were represented. This may mean that informants were those with data to contribute, but also that some specific views might have been lost which would have been gained if sampling was purposive. Information about the age, sex and other demographic information about the children concerned was not provided.

Ethical approval: Ethics committee approval was gained and the study appeared to proceed along ethically sound lines. The issues of confidentiality generally and within group settings were highlighted.

Data analysis: The method of analysing data was suitable for the data collection method. There was no mention of respondent validation, and this can in any case be problematic in focus groups. It might, however, be useful to know if there was any on-the-spot checking of interpretations or group feedback.

Results: These represented a range of views, the categories seemed to contain relevant data and quotes from a variety of parents were used to support the findings. This suggests that the contradictions and divergent views which one would expect to encounter in a group were represented, and that all group members felt able to express their opinions. Fathers' views were also included; however because of the small number of fathers, the convenience/ volunteer sample and nature of the study the researcher emphasized that these were not intended to be generalized as 'fathers' views'.

Conclusions: These matched the results. The study did not claim to be generalizable, but it provided enough data to show depth of understanding. Like the first study, it did not give specific recommendations for practice, but the issues identified are likely to be useful to help Natalie to develop services to support families.

Many of the themes developed in the studies have links or similarities, which lends more weight to Natalie considering them.

Appraising mixed methods research

7

Scenario

Kate works in an outpatients department and has been asked to look into ways of increasing attendance at appointments, which is currently below the local target level. She has come across a range of literature on the subject, and a few of the studies which she has found describe themselves as using 'mixed methods of research' or 'mixed methodology'.

The principles of mixed methods research

Mixed methods research is usually defined as research which uses a combination of qualitative and quantitative methods in a single study (Creswell, 2003; Halcomb, Andrew and Brannen, 2009; Johnson and Onwuegbuzie, 2004). This approach acknowledges that what needs to be investigated is often much bigger than one set of beliefs or ways of generating information can handle, and that both quantification and consideration of qualitative aspects of a subject may be required for it to be understood. Mixed methods research differs from two separate studies which use different methodologies because it is one study that considers data gathered using different perspectives on a subject to provide an overall picture.

Mixed methods research, which uses qualitative and quantitative methods of data collection and analysis, might be likened to comparing the price but also the quality of something you are buying. If you are buying a pair of trousers for a six-month backpacking trip, but do not wish to bring them home because you plan to stock up with goodies to remind you of your travels, you probably mainly want quantitative information: the price. However, you probably do not really just want the cheapest thing, because it might fall apart after a week, or it might

81

look so horrible that you have to stay indoors for the entire six months. So, you actually need a bit of both quantitative and qualitative information to influence your decision about what to buy. As well as having both sets of information, in mixed methods research, the analysis of this information is integrated, and inferences from quantitative findings debated or analysed in the context of qualitative findings, and the vice versa (Tashakkori and Creswell, 2007). The data from the two methodologies therefore form a more complete picture than one methodology or two separate studies would.

A mixed methods study which would be relevant for Kate might use quantitative methodology to map non-attendance figures at an outpatients department against a number of variables such as speciality, whether this was an initial or follow up appointment, age, gender or postcode. This might be followed by using qualitative methodology in which a small sample of non-attendees were interviewed to explore the data generated in the first part of the study in more depth, with any apparent reasons possibly corroborated, clarified or refuted. The demographic information might show a statistically significant higher rate of non-attendance in a geographical area which has a reputation for housing relatively affluent groups of the population. The reasons why this might link with poor attendance at outpatients would probably merit exploration. It might turn out to be related to work commitments precluding attendance, people deciding to seek private healthcare in the time between referral and their appointment or other reasons. It might reveal that the link is not between economic status and attendance, but that there have been major road works on the route from this area to the hospital for the last year which has made the journey very unattractive. The first part of the study might also allow the development of an appropriate sampling framework for the second part: for instance, the data generated in the first part of a study might be used to identify an appropriate group of people to interview in the second stage.

This may seem so logical that you are wondering why it needs a whole chapter in a book, but mixed methods research is quite controversial. Because the qualitative and quantitative paradigm and associated methodologies are based on different assumptions about knowledge, some researchers claim that the two cannot be used together (Flemming, 2007; Giddings and Grant, 2007; Johnson and Onwuegbuzie, 2004). Those who support mixed methods research argue that the distinction between methodologies need not be absolute, and that the complementary natures of all forms of knowledge should be recognized (Fleming 2007; Johnson and Onwuegbuzie, 2004). The paradigm, or belief about the nature of knowledge, which underpins mixed methods research is often said to be pragmatism (Johnson and Onwuegbuzie, 2004; MacInnes, 2009; Morgan, 2007; Tashakkori and Teddlie, 2003). The pragmatic view is that determining what will be the most effective way of exploring the matter in question should be the main determinant of research design and conduct (Mertens, 2005; Morgan, 2007). This stance makes it perfectly acceptable to combine qualitative and quantitative methodologies in a single study if this is the most appropriate means to explore or investigate the topic in question (Morse, 2003; Mertens, 2005, McAuley *et al.*, 2006; Johnson and

Onwuegbuzie, 2004; Tashakkori and Teddlie, 2003). Not everyone agrees with this, but it is the premise on which mixed methods studies are based.

When mixed methods research may be useful?

Mixed methods research is increasingly being seen as useful in health-related research, because many of the things which need investigating do not neatly fit one methodology (Curry, Nembhard and Bradley, 2009). Kate might read a mixed methods study which explores how outpatients appointments could be improved. The method used to gather data might be a questionnaire which includes both quantitative and qualitative approaches, with some yes/ no/or tick box questions and some questions which invite in-depth responses. The quantitative questions might indicate that people value information, a short waiting time and refreshments being available, while the qualitative questions might confirm this but add that the way in which people are spoken to by staff, how information on delays is conveyed and the accuracy of this are very important, with examples of what is and is not seen as 'acceptable' described in detail. Both aspects of the study would provide useful information which, when seen together, build up a more complete picture than one method alone would.

When you make a decision about whether or not to use a mixed methods study in practice, what you probably want to know is not the academic arguments for and against this approach, but whether the paper in front of you is any good. Deciding about this really means looking at the things that make research (using whichever paradigms or methodologies are used) worth acting on, applying these principles to the appropriate part or parts of the study, seeing if the findings are integrated or inform each other, deciding whether this way of doing things is sensible, and whether or not the findings seem to be 'true'.

What is the research about?

Like all studies, the first thing to look at in a mixed methods study is what the research was about. This information might be presented in a range of ways, as a research issue, question, statement of purpose or as aims or objectives. It may include a hypothesis if the quantitative part of the study merits one. There is no one correct way for the statement of the research to be articulated in mixed methods studies, but there should at some point fairly early on be an indication that a mix of methodologies was needed.

Literature review

The things to check in the literature review of a mixed methods study are the same as for any other study, and how the literature review is presented depends on the way that methodologies are mixed. If the starting point of the study is a form of grounded theory, then a full literature review may be presented or conducted once this part is complete. If it starts with a survey of what patients consider important in outpatients departments, followed by a phenomenological study of patients' experiences of attending outpatients, then the literature review will probably be carried out first. The literature review may sometimes be split into two parts, depending on the study design. However, many journal word limits do not allow for the researcher to go into great detail about when, why and how they did the literature search, especially if they did this in two parts. While it can be useful to see when and how the literature review was carried out, if this level of detail is not given, it may not be anything to do with the study's quality, but may just mean that the researcher prioritized reporting on other things. Mixed methods means more methodology to report on, and when you only have 5000 words, something has to go.

Methodology

A mixed methods study may use any of the methodologies described in Chapters 5 and 6. Methodologies may be used either sequentially (one after the other) or concurrently (at the same time) (Creswell, 2003; Curry, Nembhard and Bradley, 2009; Mertens, 2005; Tashakkori & Teddlie, 2003). A study which Kate finds might use quantitative methodology to design and administer a questionnaire about the environment in an outpatients department, followed by qualitative methodology to explore the issues raised in the questionnaire in more depth. The quantitative part of the study would provide an overview of the situation, generate ideas about what should be explored in more depth and allow identification of suitable participants (either individuals or the type of characteristics sought) for the qualitative aspect of the study. The qualitative part would follow. Another study might start by using qualitative methodology to conduct in-depth interviews with 15 people who have not attended appointments, and use the findings to direct service development which is then evaluated using quantitative methodology to see if it has improved attendance.

Alternatively, the different methodologies used may run concurrently, and be embedded within each other (Creswell, 2003; Curry, Nembhard and Bradley, 2009; Mertens 2005; Tashakkori and Teddlie, 2003). A mixed methods study of people's experience of attending outpatients appointments might be made up of an ethnography (a qualitative methodology) and a quantitative survey. In the ethnography, the researcher might try to understand the culture of an outpatients department using prolonged observation, and in-depth discussions with key staff members and patients. The survey might be sent to all staff in the department, to identify their views on how they encourage attendance. The data from the survey could be used to capture an overall picture of all staff views, and form a useful comparison between the perceptions of staff and what the researcher sees happening. The understanding of the culture generated through ethnography might clarify why any apparent contradictions between the espoused views and those seen in practice and experienced by patients exist.

The weight apportioned to each part of the study will depend on the study aim (Curry, Nembhard and Bradley, 2009). A study might use a qualitative approach and in-depth interviews to explore how patients perceive that medical staff treat them at outpatients appointments, accompanied by a quantitative survey of all medical staff within the NHS Trust concerned. While the types of data generated in each part would be very different, they might both be seen as equally important because both perspectives are vital to gaining an understanding of the experiences of people who attend outpatients appointments. In other situations, quantitative data may be gathered primarily to generate ideas for more in-depth, qualitative, interviews. This might mean that while the quantitative aspect is an essential part of the study and must be carried out to a high standard, in the final analysis, the greater weighting or interest may be in the qualitative part. However, regardless of the weighting, every aspect of the study should be carried out systematically and diligently and have a clear place in the development of the findings and conclusions.

Methods of data collection

Like all studies, a key question in mixed methods research is: were the methods the right ones to get the type of information that the study was looking for? Mixed methods research can use a whole range of methods and they can be used in whatever combination and sequence is right for the focus of the research (Creswell, 2003; Curry, Nembhard and Bradley, 2009; Mertens, 2005; Tashakkori and Teddlie, 2003). The key question is: would this way of doing things have been a good way of seeking the information that the research question or issue required?

The data that were gathered by different methods or using different methodological approaches may be used for triangulation, in order to confirm or compare information gained from different perspectives (MacInnes, 2009). For instance, patients might be asked to complete a questionnaire which gathers quantitative data regarding how much choice they had in the time and date of their appointment, how long it took them to get to outpatients, how long they waited, how long they spent with a staff member and whether they felt the facilities were adequate. This might then be compared with qualitative data in which an observer noted whether patients were given choices about their next appointment, how long they waited, what they did while they waited, how staff interacted with them and which included some discussions with people who were waiting. The responses in the questionnaires might suggest that people felt they had no choice about the timing of their appointment. However, the observer might note that they were given some choices in making follow up appointments. Discussions might reveal that while individuals did not have any choice in their initial appointment, the follow-up appointment offered some limited choices, but only within two-hour time slots on one day of the week. The data generated from both methodologies might indicate why, while the service provider felt that they did offer patients choices, this did not translate into people feeling that they had real choices, and a need for clarity over what was meant by 'choices'.

No one mix of methods is right or wrong: it depends what the intention of the study is, and how the sequencing and use of data contributes to building an accurate or true overall picture, or a picture which faithfully represents the different perceptions which exist. When evaluating mixed methods studies, the evaluation should focus on what methodologies and methods were used, what sequence they were used in, and whether this is likely to have been a good way to explore the subject.

Sample

Sampling can be a major issue in mixed methods research because where both qualitative and quantitative approaches are used, the underpinning principles of sampling differ (Collins, Onwuegbuzie and Jiao, 2007). However, when you are evaluating a research report, the same principle applies as for all research: the sample selection and size should match the aim of (that part of) the research (Teddlie and Yu, 2007; Collins, Onwuegbuzie and Jiao, 2007). It is possible that there will be two samples in a mixed methods study, but one may be drawn from the other and they are likely to have some links or commonalities, because the study needs to be coherent (Collins, Onwuegbuzie and Jiao, 2007; Teddlie and Yu, 2007). A survey might be sent to 1000 people with the aim of quantifying their views on outpatients departments. This might be followed up by in-depth interviews with 15 people to generate qualitative data. These sample sizes seem reasonable for both the quantitative and qualitative parts of the study. It would be inappropriate to try to carry out in-depth interviews with all 1000 participants from the first part of the study, unless you had a very large research team. Equally, distributing questionnaires to only 15 people and then using quantitative methods to analyse their responses would probably be an unsatisfactory way to proceed. In other study designs, the same sample may be used across both study aspects, for example, if a survey is conducted which includes both quantitative and qualitative approaches, and is distributed to the same population (Driscoll *et al.*, 2007).

Ethical issues

The ethical issues which should be considered in mixed methods studies are those which govern all research. One specific consideration though is that participants who are involved in more than one aspect of a study should be fully informed of what each of these involves and consent obtained for each element of the study in which they participate. For example, if someone completes a questionnaire in which they are completely anonymous, but goes on to volunteer to participate in another part of the study where face-to-face interviews are used, their anonymity is lost. Their questionnaire may still be anonymous (although this may be compromised if they return it with details of their name and contact details for the second part of the study) but their interview is not. Their true identity will probably remain confidential in terms of a pseudonym or number being allocated to them, but they will not be anonymous in the way that they were in the questionnaire. Consent for one part of a two- or three-part study does not imply consent for the remainder, particularly where the implications of participation are quite different.

Data analysis

As with any data analysis, data gathered using mixed research methods have to be analysed appropriately for the study findings to have any real value (Happ *et al.*, 2006). Data analysis can be the most complex part of mixed methods research, and there is not absolute consensus on the best or right way to approach this (Happ *et al.*, 2006). This is partly because of the range of study designs and methodologies which can be used, meaning that no one approach will work in all cases. The principle is that each type of data should be analysed using the right tools for that type of data.

The data generated may be connected by the analysis of one set of data leading to the collection and analysis of another, so that while the data and analysis seems completely separate, one could not have happened without the other (MacInnes, 2009). A sequential study beginning with qualitative interviews to explore participants' experiences of using outpatients services, followed by an experiment involving sending reminders a week before appointments would probably use two approaches to analysis. The initial qualitative part of the study would probably be analysed using some kind of thematic analysis, while the second part would use appropriate statistical tests to demonstrate if there was any significant difference in attendance after the new approach was introduced. Alternatively, the data may be collected and analysed together in order to explain various aspects of one thing, albeit using different and appropriate methods. A study which aimed to explore why people do not attend outpatients appointments might include a quantitative questionnaire being distributed to all patients and staff, accompanied by a qualitative observational study and in-depth interviews with selected staff and patients. This would require the numerical data to be analysed using appropriate statistical tests, and the observation and interview data to perhaps be interpreted using thematic analysis. These data sets might not be merged as such because it would be inappropriate to analyse the numerical data using qualitative techniques and the vice versa. However, the information gleaned from both aspects can be compared, matches and mismatches identified and possible reasons for apparent differences in the findings from each dataset highlighted.

In other situations how data are analysed is more complex insofar as qualitative data are analysed using quantitative approaches or the vice versa. This can be approached by data being transformed from one type of data into another; for example, qualitative data analysed by it being coded using a qualitative approach, but the number of times codes appear then being quantified. This might mean quantification of how often each code appears within the data as a whole, or for individual participants. It may also be presented as the raw scores for each code or by calculating the percentage scores for codes to give an impression of what were the most frequently cited or important issues (Driscoll *et al.*, 2007). However, this approach does create some problems, for instance, if one person repeatedly makes a similar statement, whether this should be counted once or more than once has to be decided. In addition, the sampling approach used affects this type of data analysis, because although quantification of qualitative data can be possible, it is important that statistical tests are only applied that are appropriate for the sample and the nature of the data in question (Driscoll *et al.*, 2007). Analysing data using an approach which is not within the same paradigm as the data collection method is probably the most problematic part of mixed methods research, and exactly how this was achieved and the claims made from data whose nature has been adjusted merit careful exploration. The intention is that the data generated using dis-crete methodologies should be seen as a whole, not as two separate entities. However, it is also important to check that what has been done with the data makes sense and that where data have been transformed, the challenges and limitations, as well as the benefits, which this creates have been noted (Driscoll *et al.*, 2007).

Findings

The way in which the findings from a mixed methods study are presented depends on what methodologies were mixed, how this was achieved, and how the data were analysed. There may be two types of data presented and thus two groups of findings, and possibly a set of integrated or related findings, or a discussion of how the findings relate to and develop one another. Kate might find a study that uses quantitative questionnaires or observation to identify actual waiting times in outpatient departments, and qualitative interviews to ascertain patients' views on these. It is likely that the 'answer' to the question: 'How long do people wait at outpatients appointments?' will be presented as a series of figures showing the length of wait mapped against various demographic details, medical speciali-ties and statistics generated from these. There would also probably be a set of findings presenting themes from qualitative analysis, with quotations used to illustrate the points being made so as to verify the claims to particular findings, or to further illustrate what the researcher meant by a particular point. There would then probably be a section in which the two data sets were used to make sense of and build upon each other or to illustrate the complexity of the points being made. If any transformation of one type of data into another (for exam-ple, qualitative data being transformed into quantitative data) was undertaken, how this was achieved, and the claims made from this, should be commensurate with the type of data used. The level of significance, proposed generalizability or transferability of each finding should be in accordance with the methodological approach, sample and data analysis procedure used.

Conclusions and recommendations

In the conclusions, the study's findings should be related back to the original research purpose. The conclusions and recommendations should be an accurate representation of the full range of findings, and take into account all the data gathered, including the potential contradictions revealed by different methodologies. The recommendations made should be appropriate to the methodological stance from which they were generated. For example, the quantitative aspects of a study may provide some generalizable recommendations, while those derived from qualitative findings will probably not make this claim. Those derived from data which has been transformed from one type of data to another should be associated with claims which are appropriate for the data used and analysis process, and which convey the possible limitations imposed by transforming data in this way. The conclusions and recommendations may therefore include suggestions which attract a variety of levels of significance, generalizability or transferability, dependent on which methodology and mix thereof they were generated from.

Quality in mixed methods research

There are not many established frameworks for evaluating mixed methods studies (Creswell and Plano Clark, 2007; MacInnes, 2009; Onwuegbuzie and Johnson, 2006; Sale and Brazil, 2004). As Chapters 5 and 6 discussed, the way in which quality is assessed is very different in quantitative and qualitative studies. The question in evaluating mixed methods studies is: which set of principles do I follow? The answer is: both. The study should be a combination of whatever mix of qualitative and quantitative work it said it was, and the suggestions for evaluating qualitative work should be applied to the qualitative aspects and the ones for quantitative work to the quantitative aspects. Evaluating the qualitative element may be caught up in wider debate of what constitutes quality in qualitative research (Flemming, 2007). However, the guidance on what is good quality within each methodology should guide evaluation of the appropriate part of a mixed methods study (Creswell and Plano Clark, 2007).

One additional consideration in mixed methods research is whether the study was cohesive (MacInnes, 2009). This means whether

- the parts of the study fit together logically and usefully;
- where one dataset was said to lead to or inform another really did;
- interpretations which linked one stage of a study to the next were true or accurate;

- data transformation was not misleading; and
- any challenges created by the mixed methods approach were highlighted.

The nature of mixed methods studies is that the findings and conclusions are integrated and the methodologies inform each other, a flaw in one part of the study therefore impacts on the rest of the study, and a part of evaluating a mixed methods study is identifying whether or not this was the case.

Applying mixed methods research to practice

To decide whether or not to use a piece of mixed methods research, you have to keep in mind the intention of both the quantitative and qualitative aspects of the research, what is mixed, why and how the requisite quality standards for any methodologies used were met (Giddings and Grant, 2007). In a mixed methods study which Kate reads, the quantitative findings might indicate that patients tend to wait 45 minutes for an outpatients appointment but feel that up to 30 minutes is acceptable. From this it might be sensible to try to reduce all waiting times to less than 30 minutes. However, if the qualitative findings indicate that people value information on waiting times and facilities, and comment on things like the manner in which they are spoken to, this might be harder to apply directly, in that information and manners in speech are not precise concepts. Like all qualitative research, it shows the kind of things we should consider, but cannot exactly prescribe them. In this case, Kate might decide to implement the findings from the quantitative part of the research but with the qualitative findings in mind. This might mean attempting to reduce all waiting times to 30 minutes or less while also appreciating and acting on the importance of giving information during this time, particularly about any possible delays, and helping staff to recognize the way in which people appreciate being spoken to. That way she would have applied her understanding of what most people think is a reasonable wait, but also addressed the less specific aspects of making sure that information is given in an appropriate manner, within and after the 30 minutes.

Summary

Mixed methods research is research which uses a combination of qualitative and quantitative approaches within a single study. Its premise is that the design and conduct of research should be directed by what will be the best way to gain as full as possible an understanding of what is being studied, rather than adhering strictly to one paradigm or methodology. Any combination of methodologies and methods can be used to achieve this, but why they are used and combined in the way that they are should be clear. Data collection and analysis should be cohesive, and the quality principles relevant to the part or parts of the study in question should be applied appropriately to evaluate its worth.

Jasmine works on a medical ward which specializes in cardiology. She is interested in the number of patients who do not appear to follow the advice which they are given on altering their lifestyles in relation to exercise and diet. She is looking for more information about this, and has found the following mixed methods study:

Title: Is giving advice on dietary modification post myocardial infarction effective?

Aim: The aim of the study was to ascertain whether the advice which people who have had a myocardial infarction are given on dietary modification and how it affects their behaviour.

Methodology: The study used a mixed methods approach, mixing quantitative and qualitative methodology. The two methodologies were used sequentially with the quantitative aspect preceding the qualitative.

Methods: The quantitative part of the study used a postal questionnaire which was distributed to all patients who had been admitted to a general hospital following myocardial infarction over a six-month period. It explored whether or not they received any advice on diet, how this was provided, whether or not they followed it and why. It was composed of a Likert scale which invited respondents to rate their views between strongly agree and strongly disagree on a five-point scale. The qualitative phase was composed of focus-group interviews with respondents who expressed an interest in participating when returning the questionnaire. The aim of this part of the study was to gain a greater depth of understanding of the responses given in the questionnaire. Four focus groups were held, with five participants in two of the groups and six in the other two.

Sample: The questionnaire was sent to 207 people. The sample was derived from medical records (all those recorded as having been admitted to the hospital following myocardial infarction over the past six months), a response rate of 54 per cent was obtained. Those who completed the questionnaire were invited to volunteer to participate in focus groups. From this invitation, 30 people expressed an interest and of those 22 agreed to participate. Each focus group lasted between one-and-a-half and two hours.

Ethics: The study was approved by an NHS Research ethics committee.

Data analysis: Data from the questionnaire were analysed using descriptive statistics (percentage scores). The data from the focus groups were analysed using thematic analysis. The number of participants who used each theme was also noted numerically, to give a quantitative aspect to this part of the analysis. These numbers were expressed as percentages of the participants who made a statement within each theme.

Findings: The findings from the questionnaire were presented in tabular form showing the percentage of participants who gave each response. They were not plotted against any demographic information, such as age or gender. Findings from the qualitative element of the study were presented under headings related to the themes developed. Quotes from the focus groups were used to illustrate the points raised in each theme. The findings from the focus groups were discussed in the context of the findings from the questionnaire. All the data scored using percentage values from the questionnaire and focus groups was presented on one bar chart, to suggest how the findings from the focus group linked with or developed the results of the questionnaire.

Conclusions: The conclusions were related to the findings and drew on both data-sets to produce one set of recommendations, related to what dietary advice people are given post myocardial infarction, and what affects their views on and adherence to this.

Evaluation

Title: This study seems relevant to Jasmine's work.

Aim: These aims seem relevant to Jasmine's work and suitable for a mixed methods study because this approach allows an overall view of important aspects of the subject to be studied, accompanied by more in depth discussion of key issues.

Methodology: The quantitative and qualitative parts of the study seemed to explore appropriate aspects of the subject. They appeared to be logically linked and to form a coherent whole study. The quantitative part of the study informed the sampling for the qualitative aspect and also guided the discussions.

Methods: A questionnaire is a suitable way to gather fairly reductionist but key infor-mation from a large group. The questionnaire was not shown in the paper, so it is not possible to decide whether it actually explored the subject on question effectively. There were no details of how it was developed or if it was piloted, which affects the reliability and validity of the tool because the questions may not have been inter-preted as the researcher intended, or consistently, and may not have captured the most important points about the subject. Likert scales have some problems such as extreme response bias, and acquiescence bias, but can be useful in gauging the general views of a population.

Focus groups seem an appropriate way to gather in-depth views from individuals, they present some challenges but these were acknowledged. The group size was large enough to generate discussion but not so large that some people would be unable to participate effectively. Interviews seemed to be of sufficient duration to assume depth of data were gathered. There was no mention of respondent validation being sought, but this may be problematic in group settings.

Sample: The sample for the questionnaire was large enough for this type of research, and the type of analysis used. The response rate was above 50 per cent, which is good for this type of study. However, it may still mean that the results do not really show what the population as a whole thought, because almost half did not respond and the reason for this is unknown.

This method of obtaining the focus group sample was reasonable, but because it was a volunteer sample, the participants were self-selecting. This would probably mean that they were interested and had something to share, but might also mean that people who gave responses which were particularly interesting or different from others on the questionnaire were not specifically invited to participate. It might have been useful to analyse the data from the questionnaire first and then select participants with a range of views. However, this would have meant either relying on getting a good range of volunteers to select from, or questionnaires not being anonymous.

Ethical issues: The study was approved by a research ethics committee. No specific ethical issues were discussed in the paper such as how medical records were accessed or confidentiality/anonymity/informed consent. However, this may be because of the word limit of the journal, there is no evidence of unethical conduct, and presumably these issues were considered by the ethics committee.

Data analysis: The use of per cent values is an appropriate descriptive statistic for this type of data as Likert scale data are usually considered to be non-parametric (see Chapter 5). Not attempting inferential statistics was probably sensible with this sample size/response rate (although over 200 questionnaires were distributed only a 54 per cent response rate was achieved). There was no discussion of how the researcher decided whether or not to use inferential statistics. Options within non-parametric inferential statistics might have been Wilcoxon's test or Chi Square.

Thematic analysis is an appropriate approach for analysing qualitative data. Counting the number of individuals whose views contributed to each theme is recognized as a possible approach to data analysis in mixed methods studies, but the paper did not discuss how issues such as one person mentioning something more than once was dealt with in counting codes. How this aspect of analysis added value to this study was not very clear. Although it did not detract from the findings, it seemed not to add anything that the thematic analysis would not, in combination with the Likert data, have provided.

Findings: Although both sets of findings were separate, the discussion of the findings made links between these, and used the qualitative part of the study to draw inferences about, expand on, and discuss the quantitative finings. Thus, these were integrated. The value of the bar chart amalgamating all the numerical data was not clear and adds very little to the study.

Conclusions: The findings linked clearly with the conclusions. The conclusions and recommendations were made with a caveat that the response rate and data analysis method in the quantitative phase meant that the findings were not generalizable. The qualitative part did not make any claim to generalizability. The suggestion was that the study gave some useful insights and ideas but could not provide generalizable recommendations.

Jasmine could use this study's findings for exactly what it suggested: to give her some pointers about what might be worth considering, but not recommendations which she can confidently apply to every situation.

Using summaries of evidence

8

Scenario

Ruth works as a school nurse, covering several primary schools in an inner city area. She is part of a group who are developing initiatives to address obesity in primary school children. She and her colleagues have found a vast amount of information on the subject, including research papers, case reports, expert opinions, examples from practice and clinical practice guidelines. However, despite the abundance of information and what looks like 'evidence', they are struggling to decide on the most effective way to develop practice locally.

Using summaries of evidence

Sometimes when you carry out a search, you are overwhelmed with information. This can make the task of finding and appraising it all, and figuring out how it fits together, appear insurmountable. Several studies may exist which all seem to give different advice, or there may be a few studies that are 'small' or 'statistically insignificant' making it hard to know if there is enough evidence to act on. With a subject like childhood obesity, which has many possible and interrelated causes, predisposing factors, preventative and intervention options, it can be difficult to know how to put all the information together into a coherent whole. If accurate summaries of the existing evidence are available, they may clarify the overall view on a subject, and reduce the time and effort required to trawl through and evaluate each individual study.

If someone has, recently, systematically, reviewed all the evidence on the subject of childhood obesity, then Ruth is faced with the task of evaluating the review or reviews, rather than perhaps over a hundred papers. In my mind, guidance based on someone else evaluating and summarizing the existing evidence so that I do not have to seems a good thing. However, there are some issues which need to be considered in using summaries of evidence.

This chapter starts by discussing one of the accepted ways of summarizing evidence: a systematic review. It looks at what a systematic review should include, and some ways of summarizing evidence in a systematic review. It then discusses clinical guidelines, what they are and the forms of evidence that they may include.

Systematic reviews

A systematic review is what it says it is: a review, carried out systematically and rigorously, of all the available evidence on a subject. It should follow a process which minimizes the risk of the apparent findings being due to chance, error or bias (Dixon-Woods *et al.*, 2006). The key characteristics of a systematic review are

- Clearly stated objectives
- A systematic search for evidence
- Pre-defined eligibility criteria for the studies that will be included
- A clearly stated and reproducible methodology
- An assessment of the validity of the findings
- A systematic presentation and synthesis of the characteristics of the studies and their findings

(Green *et al.*, 2009)

Many of the decisions which need to be made about using the information from a systematic review are almost exactly the same as those required for making decisions about research, but some particular considerations are given below.

Statement of purpose and objectives

A systematic review should have a clear statement of purpose, or question, so that you know exactly what it is about. It will usually also have detailed objectives which clarify: the intervention or phenomena of interest, who it applies to, the settings it applies to (if that is relevant), the types of evidence or studies that will be used and what the outcomes of interest are (Hemingway and Brenton, 2009; Murphy, Robinson and Lin, 2009). One approach to check whether the objectives for a systematic review are clear is to identify what the population, the intervention, the comparison and the outcomes of interest are (often referred to as 'PICO': population, intervention, comparison, outcomes) (Bettany-Saltikov, 2010; Flemming, 1998). A review which Ruth finds might be titled: 'A Review of the Role of Exercise in Reducing Childhood Obesity', but it would also need to have specific objectives such as: 'To identify whether exercising three times a week reduces weight in obese children aged 5–11' and 'To use evidence drawn from randomized controlled trials to identify whether exercising three times a week reduces weight in obese children aged 5–11'. This suggests that

The intervention of interest is exercising three times a week
Who it applies to is obese children aged 5–11
The type of evidence is randomized controlled trials
The outcome of interest is weight loss

In PICO terms:
The population is: children aged 5–11 who are obese
The intervention of interest is: exercising three times a week
The comparison is: exercising less than three times a week
The outcome of interest is: weight loss

Having clear objectives is useful because it means that you can check whether the focus of the review is relevant to what you want to know about, and can evaluate whether the reviewers provided evidence which was clearly focused on the stated areas. You can also use the objectives to see whether it is likely that the review will have missed important evidence which did not meet its criteria. For example, relying solely on the above review would exclude evidence from anything other than Randomized Controlled Trials (RCTs), which might mean that important evidence was missed.

Search strategy

For a systematic review to earn its name, it has to be a review of all the relevant evidence: and to be certain of achieving this, the evidence has to be searched for systematically. In order for readers to make a judgement about whether or not this was achieved, the review should detail how information was sought (Bettany-Saltikov, 2010; Green *et al.*, 2009; Hemingway and Brenton, 2009; Murphy, Robinson and Lin, 2009). The keywords and combinations of keywords that were used in the search should be listed somewhere in the review so that the reader can decide whether these would be likely to identify all the relevant information (Murphy, Robinson and Lin, 2009). If a systematic review about screening for childhood obesity stated that the terms 'obesity' and 'childhood' were the only ones used in the search, papers which used the terms 'children' or 'young people', in place of 'childhood' and which used the term 'overweight' rather than 'obese' might have been missed.

The review should also state where information was sought. Although searching electronic databases is a key part of any search strategy, it can miss important information. A really systematic search includes manual searching, for example, of recent specialist publications and checking key references which have been obtained from other articles. Unpublished material, such as institutional or technical reports, working papers, conference proceedings, local policies and protocols or other documents which will not appear in searches of published academic literature (often referred to as 'the grey literature') should also be sought. This level of searching is necessary so that the reviewers can be as certain as possible that they have all the information that exists on the subject (Lefebvre, Manheimer and Glanville, 2009; Murphy, Robinson and Lin, 2009).

Whether English and non-English language sources were considered in a review is also relevant (Lefebvre, Manheimer and Glanville, 2009). Not all reviews have the resources or funding for translation, but limiting the language options can affect the evidence gathered. If language limitations were imposed on a review, it is useful to know what effect this might have had. For example, if only English-language papers could be considered, but a systematic and rigorous search only produced English-language publications, then it does not really matter. On the other hand, if this meant that six large studies were excluded, then vital evidence may be missing from the review.

It is not so much the number of studies included in a review which matters, but whether it seems likely that the search will have located all, or nearly all, the relevant information.

Eligibility criteria

Although the search should identify all the potentially relevant studies for a review, they may not all turn out to be suitable for inclusion. To decide on the quality of the review, you need to know how the reviewers decided which of the studies that they found would be included. The eligibility criteria, or inclusion and exclusion criteria, for the review should tell you one part of this (Hemingway and Brenton, 2009; Murphy, Robinson and Lin, 2009). If Ruth reads a review on strategies for preventing obesity in primary school children, it might have the inclusion criteria of children aged 4–11 and exclusion criteria of anyone below age four and above age 11. The search which a reviewer carried out might have found a study titled 'Preventing Childhood Obesity' but if, on closer examination, it was a study about 12–16 year olds, it should be excluded from the review.

In some reviews, information on a specific population or intervention is extrapolated from a range of studies to build up a better understanding of a subgroup of the population, or a particular aspect of an intervention (Deeks, Higgins and Altman, 2009). A review regarding the measurement of BMI of children of Chinese origin might well include some papers which studied a whole cross section of children. This is acceptable, provided that the results related to children of Chinese origin were extrapolated from the rest of the data in those studies, and only the data related to children of Chinese origin were used in the review. In that situation there should be evidence that only the data which met the inclusion criteria (children of Chinese origin) were used, even though this was drawn from studies which included a broader population.

Methods

Knowing whether all the available and relevant evidence was included in a review is all very well, but it is also necessary to know if it was good enough evidence to warrant any attention being paid to it. The next step of a review therefore concerns making decisions about the quality of the information which was gathered. The methods which were used to assess the quality of studies should clarify how this was achieved (Hemingway and Brenton, 2009; Murphy, Robinson and Lin, 2009).

Exactly how evaluating the quality of studies is approached in a systematic review depends on the type of studies included in the review. Generally though, research should be assessed for its methodological quality using an appropriate framework for the type of study in question (Hemingway and Brenton, 2009). The principles outlined in Chapters 4–7 on evaluating research are the kind of things reviewers look for, but to ensure that the quality of studies is consistently and reliably assessed by all the reviewers involved, a checklist is usually used. This may be an existing tool such as the CASP tools (available at http://www.sph. nhs.uk/what-we-do/public-health-workforce/resources/critical-appraisals-skills-programme), or a tool developed by the project team. The quality of the studies should ideally be independently reviewed by at least two people to reduce the chance of errors or bias in the review process influencing the recommendations made (Murphy, Robinson and Lin, 2009).

During the process of the review, the reviewers are likely to come across questions about the studies which they have, or leads to other possible data. The intention of a systematic review is to find all the existing evidence on a subject, not to critique publications for its own sake, so it is not only permissible, but important, for the reviewers to contact the researchers to seek additional information where relevant. The reviewers might contact the researchers who carried out a large study of children aged 4–11 but which did not specify the ethnicity of those involved, to see if they have separate data for children of Chinese origin. If the researchers were able and willing to supply this data, it would be remiss not to include it just because it was not specified in the original report.

Studies which are deemed to be of poor quality (as defined by the evaluation criteria for the review in question) are usually excluded from the summary of evidence, and the recommendations arising from this. Their exclusion, and how the reviewers decided what the quality cut-off point was should be documented though, so that the reader knows that they were not missed out, and why the evidence from them was not included (Hemingway and Brenton, 2009).

Findings

The findings from the individual studies included in a review are usually recorded separately, and then synthesized to provide a meaningful whole. The findings should be collated in a manner appropriate to what is being investigated and the types of studies used to produce an overall statement about the composite evidence. This might be a statement about the effectiveness of a drug, intervention or screening measure, or a summary of the main themes about a certain subject.

Two of the most commonly used ways of collating the findings from across studies and summarizing data are meta analysis and meta synthesis (both explained later in the chapter). Meta analysis deals with quantitative data, and in particular randomized controlled trails, and processes such as meta synthesis deal with qualitative data (Hemingway and Brenton, 2009).

Conclusions

As with all research, the conclusions or recommendations from a systematic review should match the data presented in the findings, and proceed logically from these. They should also be appropriate to the type of data in question (Bettany-Saltikov, 2010; Hemingway and Brenton, 2009).

As well as looking at these general points to evaluate a systematic review, the way in which data from all the studies were summarized should be evaluated. Summarizing the findings is often achieved using either meta analysis or meta synthesis.

Meta analysis

Meta analysis is a method of summarizing quantitative data from two or more studies where the outcome measures involved are identical, using statistical methods (Crombie and Davies, 2009; Deeks, Higgins and Altman, 2009). Meta analysis usually uses data from Randomized Controlled Trials, although there is discussion about whether non-randomized data can be used (Crombie and Davies, 2009; Deeks, Higgins and Altman, 2009). When meta analysis is not a suitable approach to summarizing quantitative data, other approaches such as narrative synthesis can be used.

Narrative synthesis uses subjective (rather than statistical) methods to synthesize the findings from across studies. Although this may be achieved in different ways, depending on, among other things, the type of data being used and the aims of the review, the process followed should be systematic (Deeks, Higgins and Altman, 2009; Rodgers et al., 2009). Some approaches to, and principles which should guide the conduct of, narrative synthesis for quantitative data have been developed (Rodgers et al., 2009).

Meta analysis can, if carried out appropriately, give a more precise estimate of the effect of an intervention than the individual studies included in the analysis can (Deeks, Higgins and Altman, 2009). By combining data from across studies, meta analysis effectively increases the sample size. If three studies exist which evaluate the effectiveness of 20 minutes of exercise three times a week on child-hood obesity, with 50 participants each, combining the data would increase the 'sample' to 150 (which is more likely to create the opportunity for significance in the findings). Combining data from studies using meta analysis is not actually as simple as that, but meta analysis allows for greater certainty about the extent of the benefit (or harm) which is likely to be derived from an intervention.

Meta analysis should follow the principles of any systematic review in terms of having a clear focus, searching diligently for all the relevant information, having defined inclusion and exclusion criteria, checking the quality of studies, extracting the data from individual studies and then synthesizing them.

Synthesizing data in meta analysis

Once the data and findings from all the studies included in the meta analysis have been extracted, they need to be presented as a composite whole. There is no one correct method for analysing data in meta analysis: a range of statistical tests are used, depending on the nature of the data and the aim of the analysis (Deeks, Higgins and Altman, 2009). However, the principle is that appropriate statistical methods should be used to see how confidently a recommendation for using a particular approach can be made.

The results of RCTs (which are the type of study most commonly used in meta analysis) often show the difference between outcomes for an intervention group and a control group. In meta analysis these are usually presented as ratios of the frequency of events in the intervention group compared to the control group, using the odds ratio, or the (relative) risk ratio.

An odds ratio concerns the odds, or chance, of something happening (Burton, 2004). An odds ratio of 2 for obesity in a group that exercised compared with a group that did not means that those who exercise are twice as likely to be obese as those who do not. An odds ratio of 1 indicates no association between the factor of interest in the intervention group compared to the control group. An odds ratio of 1 for obesity in the group that exercised compared with the group that did not would indicate that there is no difference between those exercising and those not doing so. An odds ratio of 0.5 suggests a 50 per cent reduction in the factor of interest in the intervention group compared with the control group. An odds ratio of 0.5 for obesity in the group that exercised compared with the group that did not means that those exercising are 50 per cent less likely to be obese (that would prob- ably be the result the researchers expected) . A relative risk ratio is about the relative risk of something happening, expressed as a ratio. A relative risk ratio of 2 implies that the outcome of interest (for example weight loss) happens twice as often in the intervention group as in the control group (Crombie and Davies, 2009).

The usual way of displaying the data from the studies included in a meta analysis is by using a Forest plot (Crombie and Davies, 2009). Essentially, on a Forest plot, the findings from all the studies in the meta analysis are shown as individual squares, and the diamond shows what the meta analysis has found to be the overall result. In more detail: the Forest plot displays the findings from each individual study as a block or square showing the odds ratio or relative risk ratio. The size of the square is proportional to how precise the study is, and the confidence intervals for the study are represented by a horizontal line from the squares (usually these show the 95 per cent confidence level: for confidence levels and limits see Chapter 5). The aggregate effect size obtained by combining all the studies is usually displayed as a diamond, with the confidence interval shown by the lateral tips of the diamond. (again usually this is the 95 per cent confi- dence level) (Deeks, Higgins and Altman, 2009). Figure 8.1 shows an example of a Forest plot. The studies shown as black squares have various odds ratios, and the finding from aggregating all the studies (shown by the white diamond) is an odds ratio of about 0.5–0.6. Because the outer edges of the diamond are the 95 per cent confidence limits, it means that there is 95 per cent confidence that for the population as a whole the odds ratio is between 0.5–0.6.

The findings from a meta analysis are only as good as the studies included and the analysis of them, and combining several sets of seriously flawed or biased

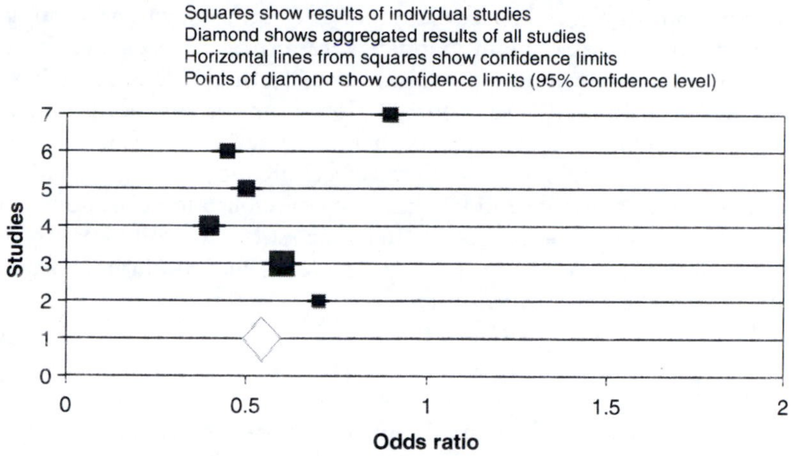

Squares show results of individual studies
Diamond shows aggregated results of all studies
Horizontal lines from squares show confidence limits
Points of diamond show confidence limits (95% confidence level)

Figure 8.1   Diagrammatic representation of a Forest plot

data will create worse flaws or biases. As well as the standards applied to evaluating individual pieces of quantitative research, some specific techniques which may be discussed in meta analysis in relation to increasing the chances of it being a 'good meta analysis' are given below.

Tests for publication bias

Because meta analysis treats the data from all the existing studies on a subject as one data set, it is important to know whether absolutely all the existing data has been included. Four studies might be used in a meta analysis looking at the effect of 20 minutes exercise three times a week on childhood obesity. The first might show that children who exercise are 50 per cent less likely to be obese, the second that children who exercise are 40 per cent less likely to be obese, the third that children who exercise are 60 per cent less likely to be obese and the fourth that children who exercise are 10 per cent more likely to be obese. If study four was missed in the search for information, then the recommendations might be very different from what they would be if it was included.

One part of trying to ensure that all the evidence is included is performing a thorough search, including the grey literature. Research that obtains negative findings (that is, ones that show no benefit from an intervention) is less likely to be published than those that describe interventions that are effective (Crombie and Davies, 2009; Moreno *et al.*, 2009) (a form of publication bias). This means that the unfavourable or neutral outcomes (such as study four) are not so often seen in the published literature: study four would be the least likely to be published. However, it is just as important to have this data in the meta analysis if an accurate recommendation is to be produced. The problem is: if you do not have study four, how do you know if there is a study four out there waiting to be found?

Searching outside the published literature goes some way to addressing this. In addition, some statistical and graphic procedures have been used to try to ascertain whether there might be missing data in the evidence that has been collated. These include the use of funnel plots, contour enhanced funnel plots (Moreno *et al.*, 2009), statistical tests such as Egger's regression test and the 'trim and fill' procedure (Duval and Tweedie, 2000a, b). However, while these and other methods attempt to address the issue of publication bias, none of them is perfect (Vevea and Woods, 2005). It is impossible to really know whether publication bias exists, but there should be evidence that the authors of a review considered it, and attempted to address it.

Heterogeneity

My son recently asked me how big the secondary school near his grandparents' home is. It has about 1400 pupils, compared to the 200 or so at his school. I figured that 1400 was a big number for a five-year old, and said that there were about seven times as many pupils as there are at his school. He looked at me quizzically, and I made the fundamental error of assuming he did not understand. 'It's like seven sets of your school', I said brightly, in the way that adults do when they are simplifying something for the supposed benefit of small children. He regarded me for a moment, with the special look which children reserve for adults who are being more foolish than usual, and asked, 'Are there seven Miss Ryves in that school then?' I had to admit that there were not. 'Are there seven Mrs. Brownings?' I had to confess that this was not the case. So it went on, through seven Huxleys, seven Delights etc until I was forced to admit that there were not seven exact copies of any of his teachers or friends there. In fact, there was no Reception class. It was just the number of children that I meant. 'So, it's not actually like seven sets of my school is it?' He clarified: 'It's just a very big school.'

Meta analysis should not include the error I made, of saying that because two studies include the same general things (children and teachers, for example) they are directly comparable. Only data that looked at exactly the same thing, in the same way, should really be treated as one set of data. It is quite unusual, though, for two studies to investigate exactly the same thing in precisely the same way, so the decision is more along the lines of: 'how different are they', and, (more importantly) 'does it matter?' The extent to which this is the case is described as the heterogeneity of the studies (how different the studies are).

There are at least three ways in which studies may exhibit heterogeneity: the mistake I made was over what would be termed clinical heterogeneity: variations in the participants, interventions and outcomes studied (Deeks, Higgins and Altman, 2009). There is also methodological heterogeneity (Deeks, Higgins and Altman, 2009): variability in study design. You might wonder how, if the inclusion and exclusion criteria were strict and have been enforced, heterogeneity could be a problem, because studies which were different enough for it to matter would have been excluded. However, the reviewers did not carry out the studies, and it can be difficult to see from the reports, even very full reports, exactly what happened. So, precisely how much heterogeneity there is between studies is not always easy to determine.

How much the above two types of heterogeneity matter is described as the statistical heterogeneity (often statistical heterogeneity is referred to simply as the heterogeneity)? This usually shows as the results from across studies being more different from each other than you would expect to happen because of chance alone. The Forest plot which shows the results of the meta analysis will often alert reviewers to the possibility of statistical heterogeneity. In the example above the way study four looks on the Forest plot might make the reviewer wonder if it was actually quite different in some way from the other studies because the results are so different. There are also various statistical procedures which test for whether heterogeneity is present, such as Cochrane's Q test (however, this test is not completely reliable) (Crombie and Davies, 2009; Groenwold *et al.*, 2010). Another test, The I^2 statistic, moves the focus away from testing whether heterogeneity is present, to assessing its impact on the meta analysis (not so much whether it exists as whether it matters) (Crombie and Davies, 2009; Deeks, Higgins and Altman, 2009). It is usually presented as the I^2 index: the percentage of the variation across studies that is likely to be due to heterogeneity rather than chance. This is accompanied by estimates of how much effect the heterogeneity matters. Crombie and Davis (2009) suggest that 25 per cent corresponds to low effect from heterogeneity, 50 per cent to moderate and 75 per cent to high, while Deeks, Higgins and Altman (2009) suggest that 0 to 40 per cent might not be important; 40 to 60 per cent may represent moderate heterogeneity, 50 to 90 per cent may represent substantial heterogeneity; and 75 to 100 per cent may represent considerable heterogeneity. However, it has been suggested that this test also needs to be interpreted cautiously, because the importance of heterogeneity depends on a number of factors, not all of which are captured by the I^2 index (Deeks, Higgins and Altman, 2009).

If statistical heterogeneity exists, the reviewer has to decide what to do about it. Removing a study just because it has different results from the rest to 'resolve' heterogeneity is not the idea: that is a bit like taking out the results you do not like. The first option is to find out why it exists, for example by reviewing whether all the studies really did meet the inclusion and exclusion criteria, and whether there are any sampling or methodological issues which could account for it. It may be sensible to consider not using meta analysis as the way to summarize the data if there is uncertainty that this is the right way to proceed or over whether the data being combined are accurate or really comparable (Deeks, Higgins and Altman, 2009). However, if you are reading the meta analysis, the chances are that that decision was not taken.

The degree of heterogeneity guides which statistical tests should be performed on the aggregated data. If heterogeneity is not present, (the studies all come close enough to looking at the same thing), then fixed-effects modelling (with statistical tests such as fixed effect meta regression) can be used to analyse the pooled data. This approach assumes that any variation between studies is only due to chance because the people involved and study design were all 'the same'. If statistical heterogeneity is present then random-effects models (such as random effects meta regression) may be used instead (Crombie and Davies, 2009).

If you are the person deciding whether the review is good enough to use, rather than the one carrying out the review, you would probably want to know whether the reviewers considered heterogeneity, whether they took some of the steps above to detect it, and if statistically significant heterogeneity was present, whether they did something that seemed appropriate, or justified what they did because of it.

The certainty of the findings

Sensitivity analysis is used to determine how the results of a meta analysis would be affected if certain aspects of the review changed, for example if a certain category of studies was excluded (such as the smaller studies or data which came from unpublished sources) (Crombie and Davies, 2009). A meta analysis of the effects of eating five a day of fruit and vegetables on childhood obesity might use sensitivity analysis to check the effects of removing an unpublished study from the analysis. If removing one unpublished study significantly changes the findings of the analysis, it could suggest that other unpublished studies being omitted would be very important, and more effort may be directed towards making absolutely sure that nothing has been missed (Deeks, Higgins and Altman, 2009). When sensitivity analyses show that the overall result and conclusions are not affected by the different decisions that could be made during the review process, the results of the review can be regarded with a fairly high degree of certainty, because nothing would change them.

In summary then, checking the quality of a meta analysis means thinking about whether all the existing data on the subject really were obtained and used, if the degree of heterogeneity between the studies was considered, whether the right type of statistical analysis was used, what the findings were, whether a sensitivity analysis was performed and whether the recommendations and conclusions seem to proceed logically from the findings.

Meta synthesis

The differences in the principles which underpin qualitative and quantitative research mean that using the same approach to synthesizing the findings from studies that use these two paradigms is not possible (Dixon-Woods *et al.*, 2006). Meta analysis uses statistical procedures, which would not be a suitable way to deal with qualitative data. The umbrella term which is often used for the processes of synthesizing qualitative data is meta synthesis.

Under the broad umbrella of meta synthesis several different techniques exist (in the same way that many different ways of generating and analysing qualitative data exist), such as meta ethnography, critical interpretative synthesis, meta-narrative and thematic synthesis (Barnet-Page and Thomas, 2009; Sandelowski,

2004). The general principle of meta synthesis though is to use the data from more than one study in order to develop, enlarge or broaden understanding of the phenomenon under investigation (Nelson, 2002). Meta-synthesis does not usually aim to increase generalizability, but aims to gain more perspectives, provide a broader and deeper view and increase the depth of understanding of a phenomenon (Beck, 2002). However, Thorne *et al.* (2002) suggest that in qualitative enquiry, in general, there is a tendency to reduce experiences into single overarching themes or patterns so that these can be neatly stated, rather than attempting to convey their complexity. This applies equally to meta syn-thesis, where the risk of findings being reduced to succinct themes is perhaps even higher as there are more data. Some qualitative researchers argue that it is inappropriate to carry out such syntheses. The counterargument to this is that unless qualitative data are presented in this form, the increasing drive to use summaries of the available evidence may erode the importance of qualitative enquiry (Sandelowski and Barroso, 2002; Sandelowski, 2004).

While quantitative researchers have a fairly commonly agreed way of analysing and communicating the findings from individual studies, and relative agreement on what constitutes study quality, qualitative researchers do not. This can be problematic when it comes to deciding how to carry out qualitative meta synthesis (Dixon-Woods *et al.*, 2006; Sandelowski and Barroso, 2002). There are, however, often described as being two broad types of meta synthesis: integrative (or aggre-gative synthesis) and interpretive synthesis.

Integrative synthesis, also known as aggregative synthesis (Dixon-Woods *et al.*, 2006) as its name suggests, aggregates, combines or amalgamates data: themes or categories which are deemed to have the same meaning are aggregated across studies. Because the aim is to pool data, the phenomena studied and approaches to data collection and analysis in all the studies that are included need to be basi-cally comparable (Dixon-Woods *et al.*, 2005). This type of synthesis often aims to develop theories of causality, and may also include claims about generaliz-ability. While this may be considered problematic in relation to the underpinning philosophy of qualitative work, if this is the intention of the review, it is really the decision of the individual reader as to whether or not they would use this type of evidence.

Interpretive synthesis does not aim to aggregate data, but to develop new, deeper or more expanded theory (Dixon-Woods *et al.*, 2005). This approach does not aim to summarize data from all the studies, and does not intend to generalize the findings: new or enhanced meanings are sought rather than con-formation of existing theory. Some people might argue that this is closer to the philosophy of qualitative work. Again, your philosophical stance and whether you would use this type of evidence is up to you, not me.

The processes for systematic review apply to meta synthesis in terms of the synthesis having a clear focus, being informed by a systematic search of the literature, decisions being made about which studies should and should not be included in the synthesis (eligibility, or inclusion and exclusion criteria), using an appropriate tool to determine the quality of the studies, analysing and synthesizing the findings, and presenting the conclusions derived from the synthesis (Dixon-Woods *et al.*, 2006).

One specific issue in qualitative meta synthesis is how to select which studies to use. Unlike meta analysis, where the intention is to find all the research which examines the same thing in the same way, the aim of a meta synthesis, particularly interpretative synthesis, is to broaden and deepen understanding. This may mean using studies which lead on from each other, take up a key point from each other, or develop what another study has done. It may be harder to decide whether all the available evidence has been used, because depth of enquiry as well as inclusion of all the studies that are available and might be relevant is important. It may also be necessary for the inclusion or exclusion criteria to alter as the study progresses, theory is developed and leads are followed. However, the decisions about selection of studies should be clear, logical and within the ethos of the review (Dixon-Woods *et al.*, 2006).

Whether the same approach to qualitative enquiry should be used in all the studies included in review is also debated. Some qualitative meta syntheses incorporate the findings of studies using different qualitative methodologies (Sandelowski and Barroso, 2002; Nelson, 2002). However, the consensus tends to be that using a combination of studies that have the same or closely related methodologies is likely to give a more coherent theoretical interpretation than that derived from the synthesis of findings from various different methodologies (Estabrooks, Field and Morse, 1994; Schreiber, Crooks and Stern, 1997; Zimmer, 2006). Neither is absolutely right or wrong, it depends on what the intention of the synthesis is, and how the differences in methodology really affect the ability to synthesize the findings.

The process of qualitative meta synthesis involves extracting or exploring the themes, findings or conclusions in the existing studies and forming these into a coherent whole. This may be achieved in much the same way that all qualitative analysis is carried out: by developing ways of identifying and displaying common ideas, codes, themes or categories across studies, and explaining how they have been developed or aggregated. As with meta analysis, it may be necessary for the person undertaking the synthesis to seek additional data from the researchers in order to get as close an understanding of the findings and as much depth of information as possible. It may also be useful to use mechanisms such as triangulation, an audit trail and evidence of negotiated validation among the reviewers as quality indicators in a meta synthesis. This process of data collection, analysis and synthesis is followed by a discussion of the meaning, implications or significance of the findings (Bush, 2002).

Given the many possible permutations on how qualitative data is handled in meta synthesis, the essential checking is perhaps that

- there is a clear description of what the synthesis was about,
- a reasoned explanation for the choices made for inclusion and exclusion of studies,
- established or reasoned and reasonable criteria were used for evaluating the studies,

- the processes used appeared to be systematic,
- there is enough contextual detail to enable you to make a decision about using the synthesis and
- all the studies included seem to have been represented in the final analysis, including those which report differing perceptions.

Mixed methods synthesis

Chapter 7 discussed the increasing use of mixed methods research in healthcare. In the same way, systematic reviews which use both qualitative and quantitative data are recognized as potentially useful in highlighting the full picture of influences on healthcare provision (Hemingway and Breeton, 2009). The quantitative evidence regarding prevention and management of childhood obesity might point strongly to a diet which includes five portions of fruit or vegetables a day and 20 minutes of physical activity three times a week. However, it is likely to be necessary to understand the quality of life factors associated with the practicalities of this in order to make it a user friendly reality for many families.

Mixed methods synthesis, like mixed methods research, aims to use a combination of all the relevant types of evidence on a subject, and to use the appropriate type of analysis for each. The assessment of review quality, like evaluation of mixed methods research, involves evaluating each aspect of the review against appropriate criteria for the methodology in question. While different processes will be used for qualitative and quantitative elements, for the review to use mixed methods rather than being two separate reviews, these ultimately need to be integrated. This may be by presenting the findings separately, but with links made between the two, by integrating them so that one set of data develops or enhances the other, or by transforming data from qualitative to quantitative for the purposes of analysis (see Chapter 7). The important thing is that there is a relationship between the datasets, but that data are not analysed using inappropriate mechanisms or processes, and that the claims made are commensurate with the type of data and analysis processes used.

Systematic reviews, then, are composed of a systematic analysis of the available evidence on a subject. They may use meta analysis, narrative synthesis, meta synthesis, mixed methods synthesis or other types of analysis and synthesis, but the processes should be clear, systematic and rigorous, and the way they deal with data appropriate to the type of data used.

Clinical guidelines

Clinical guidelines are recommendations, based on the best available evidence, about what is considered to be the most appropriate treatment and care for most people with specific diseases or conditions (National Institute for Health and Clinical Excellence, 2009). They present summaries of the evidence but also state its clinical application (Thompson *et al.*, 2001). Good quality clinical guidelines are really therefore a specific type of review: they usually include, or are based upon, a systematic review of the current best evidence, and may include meta analysis, meta synthesis or mixed methods synthesis, but also other forms of evidence where appropriate, and outline what should be done in practice because of the evidence. They often concern more than one intervention and consider a whole care package, pathway or set of options for an individual with a specific condition. In this way, they aim to give a clear indication of what should be done in practice, which can be helpful in overcoming the frequently cited problem with research of '... but how can I use this information in practice?' The Scottish Intercollegiate Guidelines Network (SIGN) have produced a guideline on the Management of obesity (SIGN, 2010) which includes guidance for management of obesity in children. Ruth might find this review very useful.

Like everything else, a guideline is only as good as the information in it and the way in which that information has been interpreted and presented. A clinical guideline which provides a high-quality systematic analysis of all the available evidence, how this relates to patient or carer experience and presents this in a logical sequence accompanied by details of its practical application is likely to be very useful. However, a guideline which provides no more information than what should be done is less useful because you have no idea about the basis on which you should do this. Many guidelines overcome the problem of 'information is great but I also need a quick step-by-step guide for everyday practice' by providing both. In the UK, the SIGN and National Institute for Health and Clinical Excellence (NICE) both publish numerous guidelines which generally include both these options.

Clinical guidelines often contain a greater mix of evidence types than some other reviews, because they cover the whole picture of clinical care and, where research-based evidence does not exist about a particular aspect of a care pathway, they use the best available evidence from a range of sources. The types of evidence which may be included, as well as research-based evidence, include case reports and expert opinion.

Case reports

Case reports usually report one or two cases of a particular condition, disorder, disease or situation. A case report in a clinical guideline on preventing childhood obesity might detail how a school nurse encouraged children to eat fruit. This may give tips and ideas which can be very useful for other practitioners, and provide valuable insights in areas where research has yet to be conducted, or where it may not be viable. However, the evidence from case reports cannot be used as confidently as an intervention which had been tested across a large population, and success shown to be statistically significant. Thus, case studies are often useful, but cannot provide confident 'always try to do this' guidance. They are more along the lines of: 'this might be useful to try, or to look out for'.

Expert opinion

The views of experts can be very valuable for guiding the 'how' of applying research to practice. However, the basis for claims to expertise vary, so exactly what is meant by 'expert opinion' also varies. In addition, the views of experts have not been subjected to the systematic approach to enquiry which is demanded in research; so papers, presentations or statements based on expert opinion are not usually considered to be as strong a form of evidence as high-quality research findings. Nonetheless, where there is inadequate research available, the consensus view of a number of experts, drawn from a variety of cases, can be very useful. Often case reports and expert opinion are combined, as an expert in the field will provide a case report with accompanying commentary.

Consensus expert view, where a range of expert views are expressed, is generally seen as preferable to an individual view because it is less likely to be subjective. Clinical guidelines often aim to have the best of both worlds, in that they use a range of evidence, which is collated by a group of experts in the field, and suggestions for its application made.

Hierarchies of evidence

Because of the range of sources of evidence which exist, hierarchies of evidence were developed to indicate which forms of evidence were seen as the best, or most worthy of use. Generally speaking such hierarchies favour quantitative evidence, because their aim is to be certain that what is recommended can be generalized. The pinnacle of evidence in such hierarchies is usually systematic reviews, especially those using meta analyses of RCTs, followed by highly generalizable evidence forms such as RCTs (National Institute for Health and Clinical Excellence, 2005). Other forms of quantitative research are placed further down in the hierarchy, followed by things like case reports and expert opinion. The place of qualitative research in such hierarchies has always been problematic: while there is some agreement on the importance of qualitative research in healthcare, how to incorporate it into a model in which generalizability is the key indicator of quality is difficult. One of the ways in which hierarchies of evidence are presented is by using a grading system for evidence where high-quality evidence is graded as 1 or A and lower forms of evidence allocated lower numbers or letters.

One of the advantages of such hierarchies is that they create clarity over what type of evidence is considered to be the best, and that some forms of evidence are, in principle, more trustworthy than others. However, a strictly hierarchical model can mean that inadequate consideration is given to what the evidence is for, and a suggestion that something generalizable is the best form of evidence in all situations (Glasziou, Vandenbroucke and Chalmers, 2004; National Institute for Health and Clinical Excellence, 2005). For example, it might be shown almost unequivocally from the evidence derived from RCTs that taking more exercise can be useful in combating childhood obesity, but it may be equally essential to have an understanding derived from qualitative data or case reports concerning how to work with children and families to achieve this. Another problem with hierarchies is that they deal with the type, not necessarily quality, of evidence (for example, a low quality meta analysis may be graded more highly than a very diligently performed case-control study).

For these reasons, there is now a move away from preordained hierarchies of evidence to the use of general principles to inform the development of guidance (National Institute for Health and Clinical Excellence, 2005). This approach uses the principles of critical appraisal to identify the quality of evidence, rather than grading it by type. The principle when considering whether or not to use evidence, whatever type it is, focuses on how good the evidence is, and how appropriate it is for the situation in question.

Summary

To decide whether or not to use a summary of evidence you have to decide how good a summary it is and whether or not it applies to your practice. It would seem overly diligent in some respects to decide to look out all the evidence about something yourself when someone else has done the job already. Sometimes though, if you are not really convinced about the quality of a review, or if there are a couple of points that require clarification, it may be worth going back to the original source. If the review is of poor quality it is not worth using. That said, using things like meta analysis, meta synthesis, systematic reviews and clinical guidelines, when they are of good quality, and use the right type of evidence for the right thing, can be very useful and effective ways of using research in practice.

Worked example

James manages a residential service for adults with severe learning disabilities. A number of queries have recently been raised by staff about the use of restraint in the service, and as a result James wants to develop guidance about this. What might he want to consider in developing guidance on this subject for his unit?

Things that James might want to consider

Does he need to develop his own guidelines, or do some already exist?

Has he searched the appropriate sources, including relevant databases and specialist collections such as the Cochrane reviews, NICE and SIGN. It may also be useful for him to use general search engines to look for guidelines from other organizations. If he finds existing guidelines/protocols, he should think about whether they provide enough rationale for him to know that they can be safely used. He should also check the quality of the guidance provided, using processes appropriate to the type of evidence used.

If James needs to develop his own guidance:

James will need to decide on the exact focus of his work: the eligibility, or inclusion and exclusion, criteria. This may include whether he wants to develop guidance for restraint in all situations that might affect his clients, or guidance related to restraint when violence is threatened/for essential medical procedures or other specific situations. He might find it useful to use something like the PICO tool to make sure that his aim and objectives are well focused.

If he is developing a guideline, James may want to repeat any previous searches following the development of his inclusion and exclusion criteria, making sure that he has included the right key words and phrases to perform his search, and possibly use Boolean terms to make his search more efficient. He should use a combination of appropriate databases, including specialist data bases such as Cochrane reviews and NICE and SIGN guidance, general search engines, cross check the references from information he gathers and investigate other resources which might be useful to retrieve 'grey literature', including contacting known experts in the field.

What type of evidence is he likely to find?

Knowing what type of information is likely to be available may help James to decide if he seems to have found all the relevant information and how he will summarize it. Thinking about the likelihood of different types of evidence existing (for example, whether it is likely that RCTs on this subject exist) will be useful in assisting him to feel confident about whether he really has all the information.

Although guidance on this subject seems important, there may be very limited research evidence on it. If this is the case, guidance can still be developed based on the current best evidence. The important thing is to be very clear about the type(s) of evidence used and any limitations arising from this. In a subject like this, which has legal, ethical and practical as well as effectiveness and efficiency considerations, it will be very important to have not just research evidence but the consensus view of those who are deemed to be experts in the field.

If the evidence from research is relatively weak, the importance of having a team of experts from across the disciplines involved, service user/service user representation and peer review of guidance before implementation becomes doubly important.

Putting it all together

James will need to decide on an appropriate way to synthesize the evidence he gathers. It seems unlikely that he will have enough RCTs on the subject to carry out a meta analysis. He may find some quantitative studies whose results could be synthesized using alternative means, such as narrative synthesis, and possibly qualitative research which merits meta synthesis. However, he is likely to need to carry out processes which involve summarizing the data from across non-research sources. Because such procedures do not have such clear processes to follow as, for example, meta analysis, it will be useful for him to have a group of experts to work with to decide how to achieve the synthesis of information, and to ensure that errors of judgement, misinterpretation, or bias do not affect the recommendations, and that nothing is missed.

The guidance which James develops is unlikely to be able to be proven to be effective in every situation, as would perhaps be the case in performing a meta analysis of the effectiveness of a drug. However, using a panel of guideline developers which includes expert opinions of practitioners and service users, he is likely to be able to make recommendations for best practice, and practical guidance, which can be used in his service. This should probably be accompanied by an appropriate form of evaluation to test whether these guidelines work and improve practice.

Part III
Putting research into practice

Making decisions

9

Having spent the past eight chapters talking about research and other forms of written evidence, it is now time to say that these are not enough to make decisions in practice.

Before you get justifiably enraged that this revelation is made after eight chapters of your life have passed by, this is not to deny the importance of research, and any of the other forms of evidence mentioned so far. It is that, in the vast majority of cases, the information from research alone is not enough to make a decision. Using research on its own might be like ordering one *tapas* dish. Even if it is a really good dish, you need more than that for a meal. You should still order your favourite dish, but you need to put something else with it if you want to go away well fed. Similarly, you probably need to put more than just research into your decisions about care for you or patients to feel satisfied.

What you need to make a decision

One of the reasons why research is not used as much as researchers might hope it will be is that exactly how to put the findings into practice is not always clear. You need to know whether and how to apply the 'looks good on paper' to your practice situation. Research may also seem unattractive because it is perceived to under-value the importance of experience, or expertise in practice. It can sound as if it is necessary to choose whether to use evidence from research, the knowledge gained through years of experience, or something else. The reality is that none of these are exclusive, and that, like *tapas*, you usually need a bit of everything. You also occasionally need to reach across to someone else's plate and grab a little bit of theirs.

Evidence-based practice requires a range of forms of evidence to be used (Aleem *et al.*, 2009; Di Censo, Cullum and Ciliska, 1998; Hahn, 2009; Sackett *et al.*, 1996). Assuming then that good-quality research and other forms of evidence such as clinical guidelines are available on the menu for the eventual decision, what else should be there? Information about the person or situation in question is obviously important. This includes their diagnosis; current clinical state; your existing knowledge of the person; notes which have been made about them; your own experience for making sense of this information and comparing this situation to cues, events or situations you have come across previously; and other people's views, experience and knowledge (Hedberg and Larsson, 2003). Finally, but not at all last in the order of priority, is information from the person most concerned, the patient: their knowledge, views, experiences and feelings about the situation (Aleem *et al.*, 2009; Di Censo, Cullum and Ciliska, 1998; Hahn, 2009; Sackett *et al.*, 1996).

The decision-making ingredients therefore include research and other forms of written evidence, observation of the particular situation in question, personal experience, the knowledge and experience which others are prepared to share, and the views and experiences of the patient. For the best decision, they are all needed, but they also need to be used in the right amount for that particular decision.

That is probably all that needs to be said really, but it may be worth thinking about each item on the menu a bit more.

Clinical judgement and expertise

Even when high-quality research, whose application to practice is abundantly clear, exists, you still have to decide whether it fits the situation you are in. Written evidence will never have seen or met the patient whom you are caring for, or been in exactly the situation in which you are working. Good decision making requires the use of sound or expert professional judgement. The distinction between clinical judgement and expertise is not always made, and often they are used almost synonymously. However, I suspect that they are not the same. I suspect that the real distinction is that clinical judgement can include good judgements and not such good judgements. We have all come across people who have bad judgement but use it a great deal anyway, and clinical judgement is just the same. Using bad judgement in clinical practice is probably not very helpful, whereas using sound or expert judgement is very valuable.

Although expert clinical judgement is the ideal, it is possible to make sound judgements before attaining expertise. Like most things, developing expertise is a process that develops over time and many people can make very good judgements even if they are not the expert they would like to be. Most experts also develop their decision making skills without really thinking about how they do this. However, when you are justifying your decisions, it can be useful to think about how they were made. That, rather than trying to complicate something which can happen without reading how to do it, is the reason for this discussion.

Experience

Theoretical knowledge alone is not enough for a person to make expert clinical decisions (Bonner and Greenwood, 2006; Mylopoulos and Regehr, 2009;

Nojima *et al.*, 2003). Knowing something does not mean that you know what it looks like. Knowing that a damp arterial trace might mean that an arterial line is positional rather than that the child is dropping their blood pressure is all very well, but you have to know what a damp trace looks like to make that decision. You also have to know what a child who is dropping their blood pressure might look like and what else about them would probably change, so as to decide whether it seems likely that the line, not the child's condition, is the issue. You also probably need to have seen this kind of thing often enough to be confident of your decision (Bonner and Greenwood, 2006).

Having experience provides you with knowledge about what something actually looks like, and a bank of previous events against which to compare what is happening right now, match situations and recognize patterns (Bonner and Greenwood, 2006). However, most writers agree that experience alone is not usually enough to guarantee good decision making (King *et al.*, 2008; Rassafian, 2009). Like every other form of evidence, experience is only as good as that experience and what has been made of it. Many years' experience will not create a good bank of evidence unless the right things were done in those years and the information which that experience provided has been used to good effect. King and Clark (2002) and Martin (2002) consider that for experience to create expertise, individuals must have in some way analysed and used it to refine their practice. Questioning or analysing even what seems to be successful practice can be important because it may just be luck that nothing has gone wrong.

Experience is therefore a necessary part of developing expertise, but of itself it is not enough (Mylopoulos and Regehr, 2009; Nojima *et al.*, 2003). It seems that both experience and theoretical knowledge are needed for expertise to develop, but how these are combined to make sound or expert clinical judgements is often the question (Considine, Botti and Thomas, 2007).

Putting experience and knowledge together

Analysis is often seen as a vital part of expert decision making (King and Clark, 2002; Martin, 2002). This involves analysis of the situation which is in front of you, the theory which applies to the situation, how this compares with your previous experience, and the ability to synthesize how it all fits together in this particular case (Bonner and Greenwood, 2006).

One suggestion is that expert decision-making skills develop through critical reflection (Paul and Heaslip, 1995). In order to reflect, you need experience to reflect on, but that experience, its link with other experiences, and how this compares with theory on the subject in question is also critically considered. This process forms a bank of information based on experience which directs and refines ongoing practice (Christensen and Hewitt-Taylor, 2006). There is a tendency for reflection to be seen as an academic exercise, conducted and documented away from the practice setting. There will be times when a particular situation causes even the greatest expert to think about it after the event, to look up information, and ponder what they did and whether this was the best option. However, in many cases the reflection which is used to develop and refine expert decision making becomes immediate and reflexive (Christensen and Hewitt-Taylor, 2006). The suggestion is that the synthesis of information which happens in expert decision making ultimately becomes an almost subconscious part of everyday practice. As well as knowing the theory, an expert fully and comprehensively assesses the patient in front of them, ascertains their views and preferences wherever possible, compares all this information with their previous experiences, and weighs it all up right there and then. Although the components of reflection all exist, they are so rapidly assimilated that the actions appear intuitive, not thought out (Christensen and Hewitt-Taylor, 2006).

Exactly how what often appears to be, or is labelled as, intuition develops is the subject of great debate, and not all subscribe to the reflection, developing into reflexive, reflection in action, theory. However, Lyneham, Parkinson and Denholm (2009) claim that what is termed intuitive practice develops through the joint aspects of knowledge, experience, and time for staff to be reflective. It would be forbidden to write about expertise without talking about Patricia Benner. Benner (1984) is renowned for her work on how expert nurses work and make decisions. She describes expert judgement as intuitive, but based on the ability to recognize patterns of events or situations, note similarities between situations, use common sense to understand what might be happening, having skilled practical knowledge of how things work, a sense of how important each particular aspect of what is seen is and the ability to think things through rationally. Benner's work, although much acclaimed, has its critics. The emphasis on intuition, as opposed to factual evidence, underpinning expert decision making has been questioned by Lemmer, Steven and Grellier (1998), and Standing (2007) suggests that Benner underestimates the value of theoretical knowledge, including knowledge gained from research. However, Benner's (1984) work does not necessarily displace the role of theoretical knowledge. Alongside other explorations of expert decision making, such as the work of Lemmer, Steven and Grellier (1998) and Standing (2007), it suggests that the expert decision maker uses a range of types of knowledge, as appropriate to the situation in question, to rapidly, accurately and almost subconsciously make a decision.

What is clear then is that high-quality or expert decision making requires the integration of knowledge and experience. However, as well as the knowledge and experience of the staff involved, good-quality decision making should usually involve the patient.

Patient experiences and preferences

It makes immense sense that the person whom the decision is 'done to' has some choice in it. While healthcare professionals may have considerable information based on theoretical knowledge, and years of practice, ultimately we walk away from the situation whereas the patient involved does not. It therefore seems odd that anything but patient involvement or even centrality in decision making could seem a good idea. In some circumstances patients may not be in a position to participate greatly in decision making, for example, if they are critically ill. However, where decisions which are made require input from the patient in order for them to happen at all, such as taking medication, or attending appointments, the decision actually does rest with them. If they think something is a waste of time, they will possibly not do it, however much we write it down as the decision made. Taking no notice of, or discounting, their views therefore seems foolish, because in most situations people will not have to do anything they do not want to. It seems much more logical for everyone to know what the individual has decided they will do, even if we do not all agree with their choice.

As well as this type of logic, many decisions in healthcare do not have clear 'right' or 'wrong' answers. This often means that no one but the individual who is affected by it can determine what is a good or bad outcome because that depends on their values and priorities (Protheroe et al., 2000). Healthcare staff may know the chances of what is deemed to be a good outcome happening as a result of a given intervention, and the current evidence about how people in a broadly similar situation have responded. However, they will not usually know how much any effects, side effects or duration of effect matters to an individual. Therefore, to achieve good decisions for individuals, the perspectives of those individuals must be included, and given as high a priority as possible. Sometimes, the technically correct solutions just do not work for the individual. For instance, a man who has chronic lung disease might benefit from a full respiratory assessment and review of all his medications, which would require three days worth of hospital appointments. However, if he is concerned about taking this amount of time off work, it may not be the best option for him, even though it might enable his medical treatment to be more efficiently titrated.

Respect for autonomy, or the right which people have to make self-determining choices, is one of the basic ethical principles of healthcare (Lowden, 2002). The focus on patients being involved in decision making about their health is, however, relatively recent. Traditionally, healthcare staff were seen as knowing what was good for patients, and it was therefore considered appropriate for them to make the decisions, and inform the patient of what these were (Kennedy, 2003). The reasons which have been proposed for a shift from this stance to an acceptance of the need to involve patients in decisions about their care include an increase in democratic thinking in healthcare; seeking to honour basic human rights in healthcare relationships (Gallant, Beaulieu and Carnevale, 2002); individuals being more aware of their rights and expecting to be given information and to make their own decisions (Kennedy, 2003); deference no longer being unquestioningly given to professionals (Wilmot, 2003); and the view of health as a wider concept than that presented by the biomedical model being increasingly common (Wilmot, 2003). The result is that patients' views are now generally seen as a requisite part of healthcare decision making. Notwithstanding this, the resources available for healthcare provision are finite and choices are therefore sometimes necessarily limited. This, and the reality and reasons for the limitations on choice, is a part of the information which should be available to patients in order for them to make informed decisions.

This does not, however, mean that patients should be left to make decisions all on their own. Autonomy is concerned with self-determination, but a person who is acting autonomously can seek and accept advice, support and assistance from others, and can also choose to defer to others. Autonomous decision making means that the individual has the right to a full range of information on which to base their decision, to make their own decisions, and to decide how much influence others have in their decision making (Kaplan, 2002; Lowden, 2002). Respecting patient autonomy should be within the context of honest informa-tion exchange where individuals are supported in finding the best decision for them (Orfali and Gordon, 2004). The key difference between patient autonomy and medical paternalism is that the influence afforded to the views of others, and their involvement in the decision-making process, is the choice of the individual patient, not imposed upon them.

One of the roles which healthcare staff may have in supporting people in autonomous decision making is to help them to make sense of the plethora of information which is available. The range of information which is easily accessible, for example, via the Internet, can be very useful, but may also be confusing, mis-leading or incorrect. While respecting different viewpoints, priorities, choices and patients' expertise in their own condition is vital, helping people to sift through the array of variable quality information available, supportively discussing exactly what the information means and helping them to explore the pros and cons of their choices can be invaluable. This may include explaining, and exploring with them, the quality and applicability of a variety of 'research findings', and other forms of apparent evidence.

In some situations, patients will have more medical or technical information about their particular condition than healthcare staff. It is an almost impossible task to be aware of all the information in all areas of healthcare practice. People who have a given condition often access a greater volume of more current information about it than healthcare professionals could possibly achieve (Hewitt-Taylor, 2006). The decision-making process should therefore centre on open dialogue, in which each party contributes their own knowledge and expertise, from which those most affected make a choice, but within a real-world context in which everything cannot be provided for everyone.

Knowledge, experience, the values and beliefs of healthcare staff and patients all need to be included in effective, shared decision making about what will be best in individual cases (Hu, Kemp and Kerridge, 2004). Decision making in children and those whose ability to make decisions for themselves is in question are important, but specific, considerations. The principle though is that the person or people who are affected should, wherever possible, be the cornerstone in decision making about their health.

Making the 'right' decision

Evidence-based practice requires not just awareness of all the available forms of evidence, but synthesis of them (Rolfe, Segrott and Jordan, 2008). This means making sense of the various aspects of a situation, the different views which exist about what should be done and reaching a decision which has weighed all these up, seen what they might mean in this particular situation and create what seems to be the best outcome. Sometimes this will mean that even high-quality research is considered, seen as not quite applicable in this situation or not in accordance with the outcome the patient wants, and thus, on this occasion, not selected. The question nonetheless sometimes remains over what should be afforded the most weight when the sources of evidence do not agree.

It is great when all the evidence points the same way, but often all the sources of evidence do not agree and there is no one clear winner. If the research confirms our knowledge gained through experience and expertise, the patient says they think it seems a good idea and it does not inconvenience anyone else then that is just grand. Some decisions are like that and do not give any trouble, but unfortunately the evidence which we have is not always consistent and one of the skills or challenges of decision making is to decide what gets the most weight.

The first step is perhaps acknowledging that clinical decision making is not always easy. There are some situations where it is pretty easy to decide what to do: cardiac arrest is relatively easy to decide on because there is a clear algorithm. Continuing care decisions are often harder. The reality is that for every decision there are lots of things to consider, and weighing everything up, in conjunction with those who will be on the receiving end of care, and deciding what carries most weight in any given situation, or what the balance is, is not easy. There is no replacement for an often rather messy and imprecise decision-making process. There are some things that make it easier but ultimately the truth is decisions need to be made and some are hard to make. Sometimes you will know almost at once if you got it right, but with some decisions you will never know for sure.

There are various decision-making models and aids which can be used and it may sound as if these will save us all a lot of hassle and soul searching: however even the best decision-making tools, or guides, are not decision makers. Some decision making models can be very useful in terms of providing a clear thinking structure (e.g., DECIDE, Guo 2008). For them to be useful, though, they have to be accessible and user friendly (Bowles et al., 2009). While information technology can be very useful for aiding decision making, the essential factor in its value, as with any decision-making aid, be it paper or computer based, is whether the system is good or not (Liu, Wyatt and Altman, 2006). Information technology alone cannot solve complex decision making (Jadad, 2002). Health professionals using any type of decision-making tool still have to apply their own clinical judgement to individual situations. Having said that, and while decision-making tools can only ever be an aid, if they are well designed, they may help us to think more systemically and efficiently and to remember all the things we need to think about and weigh up (Effken et al., 2010).

Every piece of the evidence that you have matters, and a good decision is a well-thought one (albeit sometimes instinctively rather than consciously thought through). How much weight is given to each aspect of the decision depends on what you are deciding. No one can prescribe that for you.

Explaining and defending your decisions

One of the things that puts people off using research is that they wonder what they will do if questioned about what they are doing, and how they will defend themselves. The subsequent chapters will discuss changing practice, and ways to make it less threatening for yourself and others. However, there is often no absolute right or wrong in clinical decision making. Although intuition and being an expert practitioner are great, and when you make an intuitive decision and it is right you feel good, being able to unpick your decision trail can be useful, because it means that you can justify why you did what you did and explain it to others. Developing ways of analysing decisions means that when you are asked why you did something, explaining what might have been very high-quality intuitive practice is second nature and does not faze you. Occasionally, you may also see how you could have done something differently or better, and learn from it.

Having said all that, if we make enough decisions, even with all the expertise we have, we will eventually make a wrong decision, but making no decisions all our lives just in case we make a wrong one is probably worse. So, we have to accept that many, if not all, of us will from time to time get it wrong. Being able to accept this makes it possible for us to recognize it, learn from it and take remedial action at an early stage. Often the decision will be reversible. While there is no excuse for very poor decision making, if enough thought has gone into a decision that has turned out to be wrong, that is not necessarily your fault or an indictment on you. Recognizing when a decision needs to be changed is just as important as any other part of expert decision making.

Summary

Research should certainly be one of the things that you consider in order to make a decision, but, of itself, it is not enough to make clinical decisions, and it should not necessarily always be the most important consideration. You also need experience, but experience which is informed and developed by thinking about and reflecting on this, the opinions of experts, colleagues and views of those on the receiving end of the decision. This combination also needs to have just the right amount of each type of evidence, and be synthesized in order to make what seems the best decision. On many occasions though there will be no clear right or wrong and accepting that decision making in clinical practice is not a precise science is essential. Being able to make a reasoned and reasonable decision is important, but so too is being aware that decisions may be wrong or that things may change, and being prepared to review earlier decisions in the light of new or reviewed evidence.

Changing your practice

10

If you have gone to the effort of finding information as described in Chapter 3, evaluating it as described in Chapters 4–8, and then deciding that there is some aspect of practice that it might be useful to change, it seems a waste of all the preceding effort not to do so. This may involve changing your own practice, or attempting to change wider workplace practice. The ways of approaching these changes have some similarities but also enough differences to merit separate discussion. This chapter discusses changing your own practice, and is followed by a chapter which focuses on changing team practice.

Changing the way you work is sometimes straightforward, and can be achieved without a great deal of effort or planning, but it can be challenging (Grol and Grimashaw, 2003). Even things which sound as if they should be easy can turn out to need quite a lot of thought. First, you have to decide whether you really want or need to change your practice. If the answer is yes, the next thing is to decide exactly what you want to change, how you can do this and how you will know whether you are making progress or have achieved your goal. This kind of logical and structured thinking can make the process of changing your practice easier, and can also help you to address criticisms or challenges, because the answers to many of the queries that your critics raise will be readily available.

Deciding what you want to change

The reality is that however desirable a change in practice may seem, some changes are possible and some are not. Before investing a lot of time and energy in trying to change your practice it is useful to check whether the change you want to make seems likely to be doable. There may be several things which you want to change, and you may not be able to do them all at once, in which case you will have to decide on what your priority or priorities are. If you spend forever juggling your ideas and thoughts and wondering what to do first, the chances are that nothing will change. Narrowing your ideas down to what is most important, relevant or achievable now, and then doing that, means that something happens. Succeeding in it may also convince you that you can change your practice, and are able to move on to the next one on the list (Wright, 2010).

Deciding what you want to change can include thinking about why you think this matters, what has motivated you to want to do it and what makes it your priority right now. Being clear about why you think it matters is useful because if you get sidetracked, distracted or disillusioned, you can remind yourself about why you thought this was a good idea in the first place. If you begin to wish you had started on another idea instead (especially if things have become more difficult than expected), it can be useful to remind yourself of why you are doing this one first. Someone else reminding you of why you wanted to do whatever it is you are struggling with, in a motivational tone, can be either helpful or annoying, depending on things like who they are and what mood you are in, but sometimes it can be useful to remind yourself.

Defining exactly what the aim of your change is means that you are clear about what you want, and that later on you can decide whether or not it has happened (Golden, 2006; van Bokhoven, Kok and van der Weijden, 2003). Having read the available literature on communicating effectively in stressful situations, you might feel that you want to change the way in which you communicate in such situations. However, it would probably be useful to decide exactly what you mean by stressful situations. Do you mean that you want to change how you communicate with colleagues whom you find abrupt and discourteous, or that you want to be able to communicate more effectively when a patient or their relative has a complaint? Knowing exactly what you mean is useful because when you come to decide whether you have achieved your aim you can be clear about your level of success. Instead of 'I think that I feel more confident about communicating in stressful situations', you can think 'I now feel able to approach patients or relatives who have a complaint with more confidence that I can diffuse the situation'. You might well find that you can also communicate more effectively in other stressful situations, but knowing exactly what has prompted you to want to change your practice allows you to determine your degree of success more clearly.

If you have decided to change your hand washing practice, it is all very well to say that you aim to wash your hands properly, but you may need to be more specific in terms of whether you aim to be able to wash your hands using the right technique, or to use the right technique on every occasion that you need to wash your hands. Being very clear about what you want to change makes it easier to decide whether your goal is realistic, what you need to do to achieve it, what progress you are making and when you have achieved your goal.

Aims or objectives

Stating exactly what you aim to achieve can be further clarified by deciding what your objectives are. It may be useful to have what are often described as SMART objectives (Doran, 1981).

S Specific
M Measurable
A Achievable
R Relevant
T Time-bound

Having specific objectives means that exactly what you want to achieve should be very clear. For example, your general aim might be 'To improve my hand washing' but your specific objective could be 'To learn the correct way to wash my hands' or 'To wash my hands using the correct procedure 100% of the time'.

The measurable aspect may not always be possible, depending on what you are doing. If you are planning to improve your communication skills, it is unlikely that you will use purely measurable evidence. You may have some numbers, for example, about the number of times you have had to manage situations when someone had a complaint and whether your approach successfully diffused a difficult situation, but the likelihood is that you will have a fair bit of unmeasurable evidence, based on how you feel your encounters go. Like in research, measurable goals in planning change are good for measurable things, but not otherwise. Perhaps more important than measurable is that you should be able to decide with some certainty whether or not you have achieved the objectives. If your aim is to improve your way of communicating with people who have a complaint, one way of assessing your success might be to decide how often you feel that you have communicated well in this type of situation. Another might be whether you feel less anxious when you encounter such situations. That is not measurable, but you do know what you expect to change, and will probably be aware of whether or not it is happening, even if it would be hard to demonstrate to other people.

The objectives should also be achievable, or at least have the possibility of achievement (Clarke, 2001; Reed and Turner, 2005). If your aim is to make sure that you wash your hands perfectly 100 per cent of the time, that may not be achievable. However desirable it is, you may work in an area where emergencies occur a fair amount and where you have to give intravenous drugs fast and without perhaps ideal hand washing. So maybe your achievable objectives are outside of emergency situations you will wash your hands exactly as per hand hygiene policy 100 per cent of the time; during emergencies a different approach is sometimes needed and approved, which you will adhere to in such situations. If you set objectives which have no chance of achievement, your plan is doomed. This is likely to be discouraging for you, and also leaves other people open to criticize your goals and achievement thereof (Clarke, 2001; Reed and Turner, 2005).

It might sound obvious that your objectives should be relevant to your aim, but the two can get separated somewhere in the process. If your aim is to improve your communication in situations where someone has a complaint, but your objectives are linked to making sure that staff handovers are effective so that complaints are reduced, that may be very helpful, but it is not about your ability to communicate when a complaint is being made. It might mean you have less complaints to deal with, which is undoubtedly a good thing, but it is not really the focus of your stated objectives.

Having time-bound objectives is also useful because it can help you to keep on track and to consider whether your expectations of yourself are realistic (Clarke, 2001). If the change you plan requires it, setting staged objectives so as to feel progress along the path to achieving your final goal is advisable. If you have two objectives associated with your aim of developing your confidence in dealing with complaints, one of which is to develop your ways of communicating, and the other is to feel less anxious in such situations, the first may perhaps be achievable in four months, but the latter may take a year. Having staged objectives can give you some evidence that even though you still feel uncomfortable when you approach people who have a complaint, on the surface you are managing the situation better, are developing your confidence and having better outcomes because of it.

Planning what you will do

Having identified what you plan to achieve, and how you will know that it has happened, the next stage is to decide how to achieve it: what you will do, and how you will do it (van Bokhoven *et al.*, 2003). This may be very obvious, but it can be worth thinking through everything you will need to do so that nothing is missed and every eventuality is catered for. If you want to achieve washing your hands in accordance with best practice guidelines on every occasion that you need to wash your hands, what you need to do may seem obvious: wash your hands properly every time. However, it can sometimes be beneficial to think things through in more detail. First it may be useful to identify what knowledge and skills you need, if you already have them and, if not, where and how you will acquire them. If a new skill is involved, it is worth considering whether you will need to practice it. If you know how to wash your hands properly but are not quite confident that this is an automatic action, do you need to practice a few times so that you can do it almost effortlessly, even when you have distractions? This may also make you faster at doing it when you 'roll out' your new practice, so that the possible barrier to your new way of working of people's competing demands on your time is lessened.

Having decided what you need to know and identified any skills you need to develop, it can be useful to distinguish when you will be learning and practising things, and when will you start your new practice for real. This does not preclude you trying to improve your practice in the interim, but when does it count: when will you say to yourself: 'From now on I will only do this the right way.' If you have set a measurable target, such as washing your hands correctly 100 per cent of the time, this is when it starts to get measured, even if only by you, and only in your mind.

It can seem very laborious to think all this through and often you will do all the planning automatically, without having to write it down, but sometimes thinking things through almost obsessively can mean that you have considered and planned for everything. Planning in detail can also mean that unexpected pitfalls are avoided. The statements of what you will do may seem quite obvious, but they can help you to keep a clear picture of where you are and where you are going, and ensure that you do not miss anything out. Thinking through logically 'what would I need to do in order for that to happen?' and noting everything that will be necessary can mean that you do not suddenly discover that what you hoped to do cannot be achieved because some crucial resource is missing.

Resources

Unless you have the necessary resources, change is likely to be difficult to effect (Golden, 2006). Resources are often seen as a concern in changing corporate rather than individual practice, but they can be relevant for both. One very relevant resource is yourself, and how much of your time and energy you can devote to whatever you have decided to do. Motivation is an important consideration in change management (Grol and Grimashaw, 2003) and your level of motivation is a very important resource to consider in personal change management. Admittedly you must have some interest in whatever you plan to do to be thinking about it, but you may need to consider whether or not it is vital enough for you to expend the necessary time and effort in achieving it. You may also need to consider whether you have the time and energy required right now. Changing your practice will often require sustained effort, and you may need to decide whether or not this is a good time to do it. Sometimes, practice needs to change immediately, but if there is scope for flexibility in the timing, it makes sense to do it at a good time. A balance has to be sought between waiting for a good time and never doing anything, but if something will probably fail just because you have too much else on at present, and expect to have more time and energy in two weeks, then it may be worth waiting, as long as you stick to the deadline and do not delay forever.

Although you will sometimes need nothing except personal motivation, time and effort to change your practice, it is worth thinking at the planning stage about whether you will need any other facilities or resources, and whether these are available (Golden, 2006; Grol and Grimashaw, 2003). Changing your own rather than corporate practice is less likely to require large expenditure or resource allocation, but even something like washing your hands more effectively may require the guarantee of hand-washing equipment. You may also need to consider whether any resources are required to enable you to develop the skills or knowledge that you need to achieve your goals. Thinking about key colleagues or others who may offer you support can also be useful. This does not necessarily mean that you want them to change practice with you, but having people who you can discuss your own progress or setbacks with, or generally rant to, can be useful.

Barriers to change

It is usually a good idea to think about what might get in the way of changing your practice: the barriers to change. These can include established habits or practice which you may have a tendency to slip back into, especially when you are busy (Grol and Grimashaw, 2003). You may also need to consider the magnitude of the barriers and what strategies you will use to manage them. If you know what the barriers are likely to be, and plan how to address them, it is likely to be less problematic if they do occur. For example, if you are planning to change your hand-washing practice, some possible barriers are

- Lack of time (Grol and Grimashaw, 2003; Oxman and Flottorp, 2001).
- Busy workload distracting you from taking the time to wash your hands.
- Busy workload meaning that you forget your resolution to wash your hands properly.
- Lack of facilities (Grol and Grimashaw, 2003).
- Peer pressure: Colleagues may expect you to move between tasks quickly which may not allow for hand washing time (Grol and Grimashaw, 2003).
- A lack of immediate evidence of harm from poor hand washing can mean that it slips into a lower priority place than more obvious demands (Grol and Grimashaw, 2003).
- Patient expectations (Oxman and Flottorp (2001): patients may expect to be seen quickly and taking time to wash your hands properly may be problematic when someone is waiting or calling you.

Knowing or naming these challenges can enable you to think about ways to overcome them or lessen their impact. For example, being prepared for the conflicting emotions of a patient calling you while you also want to wash your hands properly can help you to be ready for this if it happens.

You may have to consider how you will manage your own ongoing motivation and ability to stay with your ideal even when things do not go well. If you are a person who has no problem with sticking to a course of action against all odds, then this may not be an issue, but if not, you may want to consider this as a potential barrier and think of how you might be able to address it.

However diligently you plan a change in your practice, there is a chance that things will not go to plan. Hopefully by identifying possible barriers to change, and the exact steps needed to achieve your goals, this possibility will be minimized, but it is useful to have either written or mental contingency plans so that if something goes wrong it does not throw you completely.

Timetable

Deciding when you will start any change in practice is useful, so as to avoid the 'mañana' culture in which tomorrow is always soon enough. As well as having a start date and a date by which you aim to achieve your goal, it can be helpful to have timetabled stages along the way to help you to see what you have achieved, and whether you are on track, even if you have not completed the task yet. Sometimes you cannot set the final target date until you have achieved some intermediate milestones, so having some earlier stage goal dates can be useful (Clarke, 2001).

It is important that your timetable is realistic. Sometimes things can sound as if they will be easier than they actually are, and thinking through exactly what you will have to do to achieve your aim can help you to have a realistic and viable timetable. Any timetable needs to be flexible though: if one goal gets delayed, then the other dates will probably need to be altered in light of this, instead of you striving for the unachievable. If you find that you have underestimated the time you need for any stage, never be afraid to replan rather than trying to do the impossible.

Evaluating your new practice

Finally, you need to know whether what you aimed to change about your practice has happened, and, if possible, whether this makes any difference. This means having an evaluation strategy (Cork, 2005; Golden, 2006; van Bokhoven *et al.*, 2003). The criteria which you will use to evaluate your success should ideally measure not just whether you do something, but whether it is a good, or effective way of doing things. This may not always be possible. If you decided to change your hand-washing practice, it would probably not be possible to demonstrate that ward infection rates were affected by this: you might have to be content with knowing whether you were achieving your target of how often you wash your hands correctly. However, if your aim was to feel more confident when you deal with complaints from patients or relatives, you might be able to identify that over the past four months you have successfully diffused ten situations where someone wanted to make a complaint, and identify positive outcomes that your approach created, such as an opportunity to discuss the person's concerns, find out more details of their circumstances, and what their needs were, etc.

Planning for sustained change

Often plans for change end when the desired outcome has been achieved. However, it can be well worth planning beyond the honeymoon period. When we are doing something new, even something which is difficult and has had opposition, we can be full of enthusiasm and energy and really stick to it. However, as time goes on, we may gradually slip back to how things were before. It is worth thinking about how to avoid this and make change sustained, because otherwise the effort you put into the initial change in practice is wasted (Golden, 2006). This might be achieved by including dates at which you will check on your goal achievement far beyond the end of the original plan, for example at six months, and a year, to remind yourself of where you got to and to make sure that you are still there. Another option is to develop on from your original goal so that the same idea is taken to a higher level, or a personal project is developed into a unit project. That way, you have no real option on going back to square one.

Defending your practice

Even when it is only your own practice that you change, you may feel that you have to defend your new approach. One reason why people do not change their practice is because they fear that things will not work out and they will either be accused of malpractice, poor practice or have a complaint of some kind made about them (Grol and Grimashaw, 2003; Oxman and Flottorp, 2001). Being clear on exactly what you want to achieve, how you are going to go about this and how you will measure your success can go some way to reassuring you about this because it allows you to state clear 'checkpoints' for whether things are going well or not. If your aim is to always wash your hands thoroughly but you are worried that patients will complain that you do not see them quickly enough, then you can state (to yourself probably) that you will introduce your new practice and monitor for a week how many delays in seeing patients really occur, whether these have any adverse effects and whether anyone actually does complain. That way you have clear and defendable evidence, even if you only present it to yourself, that you took into account the likely problems as well as benefits, aimed to detect these, and found them to be insignificant or largely absent. It can be worth noting before you start your new practice, either mentally or in writing, what your worst case scenario is. This means that you can weigh up how bad that would be, how likely it is that it will happen and what you would do if it did happen.

Another important thing is to acknowledge that sometimes a good idea does not work. Not setting yourself up as a guaranteed success means that if you do not succeed, you suffer less loss of face. There is a distinction between not trying something wholeheartedly and then wondering why it does not work, and trying something with enthusiasm but realism, acknowledging that things can go wrong.

Action planning

For personal and corporate change, action planning gets a lot of airtime. There are some situations where a formal action plan is overkill. If you plan to get up 15 minutes earlier because you have a tendency to appear at work late and dishevelled, you probably do not really need an action plan: you just need to find a way to remind yourself to set the alarm 15 minutes earlier and then drag yourself out of bed. Unless of course 15-minutes less sleep is going to make such a difference that you need to get to bed 15 minutes earlier the night before and that requires a change in your whole evening schedule. Sometimes documenting an action plan is unnecessary, because you can just think things through and hold them in your mind, but in some cases action planning, or documenting your plan for change, is useful.

Action planning is really just a way of documenting the plans and processes outlined in this chapter. There is no correct way to present an action plan, but documenting it in tabular format can make it easier to remember what you are meant to be doing at a glance, see where you are, what still needs to be done and what you have achieved. Two examples of action plan templates are shown in Appendix 3.

Summary

There are likely to be times when reading and evaluating research means that you decide to try to change the way you do things. If you decide that this is necessary or desirable, one of the first things to determine is exactly what you want to change. It can be useful to start putting your ideas together on an action plan, so that you have a very clear idea about what you want to do, how you will do it, what you will need, what might get in the way, how long you expect it to take, and how you will know when and if it is done. You may also want to build in contingency plans, ways in which you will deal with opposition, and how you will sustain your new practice once the novelty wears off. You should also build in the rewards which you will give yourself when you have achieved what you set out to, or, even better, when you achieve each stage. This is why you should usually make a detailed plan with plenty of stages in it.

Changing team practice

11

Chapter 10 discussed some of the challenges involved in changing your own practice. If you are planning to change practice which involves the team whom you work with, the same principles apply, but it is likely to be a much bigger undertaking. You will have to convince individuals and groups that the change in practice is needed, and manage a range of personal and professional views and priorities concerning the change you are proposing. Because there is more to consider, it is usually necessary to think in more depth and have a more detailed plan about how to manage the process.

The process of changing practice has been likened to an ice cube melting, changing shape and freezing again (Lewin, 1951). This simile illustrates how the existing status quo is challenged, and the need for change accepted (the ice cube melting). Change is then implemented and, as the change in practice becomes established, 'refreezing' occurs. Where change involves groups, each individual is likely to be at a different stage of this process, and the ice cube might melt and refreeze in a complex or irregular fashion. When new practice is suggested, there are likely to be innovators, who initiate the change or who are keen for it to take place (those who melt almost at once), early adopters, who agree with the change and carry it forward (those who also melt pretty fast). There are also usually the early majority who adopt change to fall into place as they see others accepting it (melt, but a bit more slowly); the late majority, who initially reject the change, but eventually conform when everyone else seems to be doing so (quite late melters); and laggards, who continue to reject change and remain frozen throughout, or until the new way of doing things becomes established practice (Rogers, 1995).

This chapter discusses some aspects of managing change which involves a group or groups of people. One of the major complexities of managing corporate change is that every person is likely to be at a slightly different place in the ice cube analogy. Although thinking about the above groups is a useful guide, there is still variation within each group, so you are more likely to be managing a moving and patchy ice sheet than a tidy cube in your freezer.

Deciding on what needs to be changed

As Chapter 10 identified, it is important to decide on exactly what the aims and objectives of any change in practice are (Golden 2006; van Bokhoven *et al.*, 2003). The bigger the change, and the more people involved, the more time and effort it is worth spending on deciding exactly what you intend to achieve. It will be difficult for others to buy into your idea if you are not sure exactly what it is, and if you are not clear about what your aim is, others will not be able to decide if they would like this outcome. Having read the research about multiprofessional communication, you may decide that you want to improve communication between professions in your workplace. This is a very worthwhile aim, but saying that your objective is to instigate monthly multidisciplinary team meetings to share information and views makes what you are seeking support for clearer. It also means that you can be quite precise about what you will need, who needs to be involved, what the problems are likely to be and how these might be overcome. Another advantage of being clear about exactly what you want to achieve and why is that if the plan changes a little en route is it is easier to decide whether your core aim and objectives are still the focus (Golden, 2006).

Ways to approach change management

Chin and Benne (1985) identify three main approaches to motivating others to change their practice: the empirical rational, the normative re-educative and the power coercive approaches. The empirical rational approach assumes that people will change their practice if they can see the reason for it, and that it is in their own or the general best interests. This may be a useful approach when you are explaining why you are suggesting a new way of doing things. However, despite the importance of explaining your rationale, and however strong your evidence is, this approach alone is unlikely to be enough because it does not take into account the many reasons why people may not embrace new practice even when, of itself, it seems a good idea.

The normative re-educative approach takes into account the social and cultural implications of change and explores the reasons why people may or may not favour a new way of working. It considers the implications of change for individuals and groups, based on their culture, beliefs, priorities and values, and accepts that people need to take an active part in, and own, change for it to happen. Working collaboratively with colleagues, seeking their ideas and finding solutions which will work for them, are a part of this approach (Ludwick and Doucette, 2009). It is almost always necessary to use the normative re-educative process in whole or in part to successfully alter team practice.

The power coercive approach occurs where political or economic power is used to achieve change: fear of the consequences of not doing things in the new way drive the change, not the intrinsic worth of the new way of working. Using it may mean that the change is implemented when you are looking but not otherwise, because no one believes in it except in order to stay out of trouble of some sort. However, this approach can sometimes be useful: for example, getting influential (but not necessarily senior) colleagues on your side can mean that you have the valuable asset of peer power at your elbow. Thus, although the power coercive approach is not always helpful in its entirety, some useful strategies have elements of this type of thinking within them.

In most cases, a mixture of these strategies is needed, with each one brought into play appropriately for what you aim to achieve at the time.

Force field analysis

The discussion on how to plan change in Chapter 10 applies equally to planning larger scale change, but the more people that are involved, the more complex the plan will be. It is almost always useful to divide your project into stages or sequential action points when it is a large plan involving a whole team. This helps you to consider, for each stage: what you aim to achieve, what you will need, who will need to be involved, who will support you, whom you need to convince of the value of changing practice, what is needed for this to happen, how long you expect it will take, and how you will decide if you have achieved it. It may be useful to document this type of information on an action plan (as described in Chapter 10, and shown in Appendix 3). As a part of this, it is worth thinking about the individuals and things which may help to facilitate, or which may work against, each stage of change.

Analysing the things which are likely to act for or against change has been described by Lewin (1951) as 'force field analysis': analysis of the likely forces at play in effecting change. Barriers to change are described as restraining forces (forces acting against or restraining change) and facilitators of change as driving forces (acting for or driving change) (Lewin, 1951). For change to be successful, the driving forces need to outweigh the restraining forces so that the overall 'force' is positive. The driving and restraining forces may be related to each other, or unrelated, but the overall sum of the force needs to be positive to move change forward. A driving force for changing a ward handover process from office based to bedside handover might be your conviction that this will increase patient involvement. A reciprocal restraining force may be those who think that this will not increase patient involvement, because people will just talk about patients at the end of their beds. For the force to be positive, the combined weight of opinion (the strength as well as number of people who hold each opinion) must fall in favour of thinking that this will improve patient involvement. However, the overall force for or against this change will be made up of more than just whether people think walk round handovers will improve patient involvement or not. It will also be affected by whether people think patient involvement is a good thing (driving force), or whether they oppose greater patient involvement (restraining force), if any cost is involved (a possible restraining force), if this meets any targets which have to be met (a possible driving force) and many other factors. Assessing the driving and restraining forces that are likely to exist in relation to any change in practice means identifying all the things which might influence its acceptance.

When you are trying to initiate change which involves a whole team, you have to consider driving and restraining forces that relate to individual practitioners, groups within the healthcare team, and organizations as a whole (Grol and Grimashaw, 2003). Individuals or groups may be comfortable with some aspects of change but not others, or your team may be enthusiastic about your ideas but the wider organization disinclined to support it. Identifying restraining and driving forces at each stage of your proposed change for each group can help you to plan what you may need to do, and when you should do this.

Barriers to change

The people who will be involved in and affected by a change in practice need to own it if it is going to work (Scott *et al.*, 2003). The problem is that there are many reasons why people will be disinclined to doing things differently, and will not want to participate in, much less own, a new way of doing things. Sometimes we wonder why people oppose change, but an equally valid question is why should they accept it (Price, 2008)? It would be worrying if every time a suggestion was made everyone immediately and without question signed up and joined in.

Change can evoke a sense of loss (Price, 2008; Scott *et al.*, 2003): it can mean relinquishing security, or something that has been important to people. Seeing change as a process of loss as well as potential gain can be useful in understanding why responses to change can be negative, unpredictable and inconsistent. An individual may be seen as an expert in how something is currently done, and changing practice not only robs them of their confidence and competence but of their role as an expert: the person everyone comes to. Thus, a change which may seem to the instigator to be a minor adjustment in how patients' notes are organized can represent the loss of a part of someone else's work identity. People may also vacillate between accepting and rejecting change, for instance if they see an idea as essentially good but are not sure how they will fit into it. An important part of bringing people on board for change can therefore be to help them to find benefits, and a place for themselves, in the new way of working, in a way that outweighs the loss that they feel they are suffering (Price, 2008; Scott *et al.*, 2003).

Few of us like doing something for no reason, and people are unlikely to welcome change unless they are convinced that it is needed: how it might improve things, or even why things need to improve (Grol and Grimashaw, 2003). This may be especially so if there is no evidence of a problem. You may have research-based evidence which suggests that a new approach is better than what is currently done, but unless you also have evidence that there is a problem with the way things are done now, people may find it hard to understand why they should make the effort to change.

To make it more likely that other people will accept the change you propose and find their place in it, you not only need to explain why you are proposing a change, but to listen to other people's views (Ludwick and Doucette, 2009; Stoller *et al.*, 2010). Although it can be disheartening to have your ideas debated or opposed, not all opposition is bad. Someone voicing their opposition to a change in practice may stop something from happening which, although it looks and sounds good, is never going to work or might even be dangerous. At a less severe level, it can make you think through every aspect of your plans: you may have missed out important points or not thought of individuals who it might be useful to involve or who need to be brought on board (de Jager, 2001; Piderit, 2000; Wright, 2010). If you are suggesting a walk round nursing handover instead of an office based one, you may not have thought about involving medical staff, but discussion with colleagues might highlight that medical staff will see nurses as out on the ward and available to assist them. Involving or informing medical staff may therefore minimize interruptions and aid your project. By listening to the person who made this comment, you may discover that they see themselves as the confidante of a particular consultant. If you enlist them to tell the consultant about your idea, you may bring them on board as the one who can 'bring the medical staff round'. It will not always work like that, but sometimes listening to other people's concerns, and asking them for help to find and effect a solution can avoid problems later on, and give them a role and purpose in the new scheme of things.

Another reason why listening to exactly what other people say is important is that what they apparently oppose is not always what they actually oppose. If you are proposing a change from office-based to walk round handovers, a concern raised might be that patients will be annoyed to see a group of nurses talking (handing over) when they need something. This may in fact turn out to be more of a concern over the ward workload, and the risk of this type of handover taking longer, than anxiety about patients complaining. The concern is still valid, but identifying exactly what it is can help you to plan the right actions to overcome it.

Established practice or routines can be a significant barrier to change (Grol and Grimashaw, 2003). As well as people remembering to do things the new way, whether people accept a change in practice may be influenced by their confidence in the skills that they will need if things change (Grol and Grimashaw, 2003). Having to learn new skills or gain new knowledge is time consuming, especially when this replaces something which is currently done almost automatically. It may also be disheartening for a relatively new member of staff who has recently learnt the skills they need to have to relearn one of these. If not enough time is devoted to enabling people to learn and refine a new skill, it is likely to mean that, however good the new way of doing things is, people will fall back into old ways just in order to get things done, or because they do not yet feel confident enough to do it the new way (Grol and Grimashaw, 2003). Nobody wants to look a fool, and doing something a new way when you are confident in the old way can pose this risk. People learning a new skill often require resources which need to be secured before the change can take place. One reason why detailed planning is important is to avoid taking the trouble of trying to convince everyone about a new way of working, only to find that you will not be given the time or resources for anyone to learn how to do it.

The outcomes of new practice are usually unknown. The research may say that something will work, but often no one you work with will have seen it in real life. Even when a change seems good in theory, established practice that has worked, or apparently worked, for years usually feels safe. There may be specific concerns over liability if problems occur, or worries about complaints being made because of a new way of working (Grol and Grimashaw, 2003). A part of addressing this is to make sure that you provide enough information about how the proposed change may improve things, and ensure that if at all possible, the change is pilotable, reversible and amendable depending on clearly defined outcomes. To say that it is pilotable without saying how you will decide whether to carry on after the pilot is less attractive than having clear evaluation dates and criteria: there is often a suspicion that piloting means 'slip it in as a pilot and then carry it on anyway'. To allay concerns about what will happen if things do not turn out well or if a complaint is made, it can be useful to clarify where leadership of the change lies, who is accountable for issues arising from the change in practice, and who is endorsing it (Grol and Grimashaw, 2003). This may mean that individuals are less concerned about defending changed practice, or of the consequences of any problems falling on their heads.

People can sometimes appear to agree to your plans, but then fail to support you. This may be because they have subsequently thought things through and changed their mind, or because in the interim time someone else has convinced them of their viewpoint. This is one of the reasons why, after first presenting your ideas, it is important to have follow-up opportunities for discussion. People may never have agreed with you, but not felt able or willing to say so, or in some cases silence or agreement followed by opposition is a strategy to stop the project going ahead. People may apparently agree with you and share information and resources, but in fact withhold important information, or pass on information selectively. In the same way that it is worth checking the real reason why people oppose change, it is also sometimes worth being a little cautious of those who claim that they support you. While it is not a particularly good idea to approach change management with a paranoid outlook, not taking everything at face value is quite important. People who openly challenge or ridicule your ideas are off putting, but at least you know what has been said and by whom, and can think about how to handle it. Covert opposition can be much harder to address.

Barriers or facilitators to change may be things that are nothing to do with your proposed change per se: they may relate to other changes or challenges which individuals or groups are concurrently facing (Grol and Grimashaw, 2003). Your idea may be good, but if there have been too many other changes recently, people may need a time when they can simply absorb these and stabilize practice. Equally though, if there has recently been a successful change in practice, it can be useful to effectively ride on its bow wave, especially if it is related to your project. Alternatively, if a change in practice has recently bombed, you may want to wait until everyone forgets how bad that was before you bounce in with a new idea (Golden, 2006). A part of assessing the forces at play in facilitating or detracting from change is gauging the workplace mood in relation to new ideas.

Patient views and expectations may also be a driving or restraining force in change (Grol and Grimashaw, 2003). If you have evidence that a new type of dressing is the most effective, but the patients concerned oppose this, their opinions are likely to create a significant and possibly valid barrier to your proposed change. Sometimes patient views can feed into staff concerns, for example, patients may expect action and prescription even when the current best evidence advocates watching and waiting. This may create a feeling of compulsion to act for staff (Grol and Grimashaw, 2003), and a sense that liability is likely to be less for doing something than for doing nothing. As Chapter 9 discussed, patients views and preferences are a vital part of evidence-based decision making, and these also need to be taken into account in change management, especially when the change in practice most affects them.

Key players

It is always valuable to have someone, or a group of people, alongside you who are motivated and convinced about the change you are proposing (Golden, 2006; Saull-McCaig *et al.*, 2006). This is useful for support, to help you work with others who are less enthusiastic, and to assist with the practicalities of managing changing practice. To this end, it is useful to identify some key assistants, change agents, champions or leaders, who will help you. However, even with a group of supporters, unless a critical mass buy into the change that you propose, it is unlikely to succeed (Scott *et al.*, 2003). Thinking about whether enough people are sufficiently committed and how you can overcome resistance to change includes carrying out a 'key player analysis'. This enables you to identify who is committed, and what roles you may be able to ask individuals to take on, but also who opposes your plans, and whether the force of opinion will be enough to carry the day (Golden, 2006).

A key player analysis should include identifying those who are most affected by or involved in the change, and whether they are likely to be supporters or opponents. Perhaps most critically, it involves looking at whose opinion really counts (Richens, Rycroft-Malone and Morrell, 2004; Saull-McCaig *et al.*, 2006). The key players may be the people who are most affected, but equally they may be people who you did not expect to have anything to do with the change, but who are held in high esteem, or who voice their opinion and convince others. You may have proposed a change that is nothing to do with medicine, but if a consultant whose opinion is held in high regard derides it and convinces other staff not to take it seriously, they are a key player. Similarly, the change in practice may be opposed by one or two very influential junior grades who everyone listens to, or dares not oppose. That makes them key players. Individuals whose opinion counts are key players, and, ideally, they need to be on your side.

If the opinion leaders support you, then life is good. If not, prioritizing ways to get them on board is advisable. This may include finding out what their opposition is really about, seeking their views, and taking some of their ideas on board. If you find a part of the change that they do support, or where their ideas will be influential, encouraging them to take a leading role in that part can be useful. If, however, it is impossible to bring all the opinion leaders on board, you need to think carefully about the impact of this, whom they are most likely to influence, and how you will manage the situation so that others join you, or remain on board.

Ideally those playing key roles in change should understand a broad range of perspectives on the proposed change and be able to empathize with different stakeholders in the change process (Golden, 2006). The list of characteristics of a good change agent include: being a critical thinker, motivator, advocate, guide and having the ability to be supportive, inspire confidence and cope well with change (Stanley, 2004). You may not be fortunate enough to possess all these characteristics yourself, or to be able to engage only assistants who have them all, but having people with a mix of these types of skills and attributes, and encouraging them to take on roles appropriate to their skills and strengths is helpful. Having a number of different people playing key roles can also be useful in increasing support for your project: one person may be able to empathize with Health Care Assistants, another with medics, and another with physiotherapists. It can be useful to have people in your team who are skilled or confident in relation to the proposed change (Saull-McCaig et al., 2006), so that they can demonstrate or see how it will work in practice, and convince people by example that it is doable. Equally, a part of bringing a person on board may be teaching them a new skill first and giving them the role of teaching others. You may decide to give key roles to individuals for a variety of reasons, which may not necessarily relate to their initial enthusiasm or their ability to meet Stanley's (2004) criteria.

There is debate about whether change should come from the top down (initiated and directed by management, and required of frontline staff) or the bottom up (initiated by frontline staff). Moran and Brightman (1998) suggest that although these two approaches are sometimes described as if they are 'either or', successful change usually requires a mix of approaches. It is necessary to have those described as frontline staff on board, because they are usually the ones who will have to actually do whatever it is that the change in practice requires. So, as far as possible, those who have to 'do' the change should own it, or see it as important. However, while it is often suggested that the bottom-up approach is preferable (Pearcey and Draper, 1996; Pryjmachuk, 1996), there usually also needs to be an element of a top-down approach insofar as managerial support for any change in practice is usually crucial (Allan, 2007; Bacall, 2000). You are likely to need to canvass at both levels concurrently, creating ownership and support at both ends. However, in convincing each party that the change fits their agenda, you should be careful to remain true to the essence of your original plan. You need to be sure that you do not inadvertently sell, or agree to, two separate sets of incompatible goals. Otherwise, when the parties meet, conflict, not co-operation, will happen, with you in the eye of the storm, with two sets of plans, neither of which are what you wanted to do.

Readiness for change

Golden (2006) discusses the value of assessing how ready people are for change before attempting to implement new practice. One of the challenges of changing group practice is that people are likely to be at different stages of readiness for change. Your decisions about when to initiate change will include how many people are at each stage, what weight of opinion, or driving force, they represent and whether this means you can go ahead with implementing change or not. Prochaska and DiClemente (1992) describe the stages of changing behaviour as precontemplation, contemplation, determination to change, action and maintenance of new practice. Although Prochaska and DiClemente's (1992) work is based on changing personal behaviour, not corporate practice, their ideas may be a useful framework within which to consider your colleagues' readiness for new practice.

Precontemplation is the stage at which people are not contemplating or willing to contemplate change. They are either unaware of any need for change or are aware of proposals for change but do not want it to happen. For people to move beyond this stage they need to be convinced that changing practice is at least worthy of consideration. This may be by letting them know the evidence for change: however as well as the information itself, the amount and timing of the information which people receive can be very influential in whether or not they support a change in practice. A balance has to be achieved between information overload and not giving enough information to make something sounds interesting. When and how information is reinforced or built on also matters: it is important to keep information coming in, but also to avoid talking at length about your project on every occasion, even when everyone is busy. It is also relevant to remember the limitations of using the empirical rational approach alone, and to consider how people's priorities and values may affect their responses to a proposed change. Moving people towards contemplating change includes listening to and trying to understand why they do not see change as necessary and what might make them at least consider it.

Prochaska and DiClemente's (1992) next stage of change is described as contemplation: this is where individuals have moved beyond dismissing the idea of change out of hand and are thinking about it and weighing up the pros and cons of changing. They have still not decided to change anything, but it is a possibility. This might be a time when people are wavering, and need to hear or see more about why they should consider change, the benefits that this might bring, more detail on the amount of effort they will need to make, skills they will need to gain, and what it will mean for them. It may also be a time when having other influential people on board becomes especially useful, as they may be able to offer information or perspectives which show how things might work for individuals or for a particular group. Demonstrations of how things will work or look can also be helpful because a new procedure, form or way of doing something often sounds more difficult or tiresome than it really is: seeing it in action may be reassuring and bring someone from contemplation to supporting the idea.

Finding out what it is that people are actually weighing up in their decision is also useful: whether they are weighing up the value of what you have said the benefits of change may be, or considering what a change in practice will mean for them. 'Competing commitments' have been identified as an important barrier to change, and finding out what people who oppose change are really concerned about, be it practical, emotional or value-based is crucial to exploring if and how they can accommodate the new way of working (Kegan and Lahey, 2001). If your proposed change is to move to 12-hour shifts, someone may seem to be mulling this over, and it may be worth finding out whether they are thinking about the pros and cons of twelve hour shifts, or wondering how they can manage their childcare arrangements within this. It may be that discussing the possibility of fixed days so that their childcare can be accommodated will be more fruitful than further discussion of the benefits which patients and the organization may derive from 12-hour shifts.

The next stage of Prochaska and DiClemente's cycle is preparation for change or determination to change. At this point the person concerned has decided that change is a good idea and is on your side: your job is to keep them there. Given that people will probably be at different stages of readiness for change, when you have a number of people who are ready for change, you may well have to maintain their enthusiasm while you try to bring more people to this stage. This may be by keeping a steady stream of information going, providing updates to reassure people that the project is not forgotten, involving them in trying to convince others, and in developing some parts of the project which will be needed at later stages but which can be completed in advance. Keeping the momentum of those who are ready to change when there are not yet enough of them can be challenging, and merits some thought so that you do not lose them.

Changing practice

Once you are convinced that enough people are at the stage of determination to change, it is time for stage four: the action stage, where the change is implemented. In some respects there is not so much to say about this stage because it is where you actually do as you planned. However, at the same time as doing whatever it is you have planned, you need to keep your supporters on board, try to recruit more support, and lessen any opposition (Golden, 2006). Although you may have a critical mass who are ready for change, you are still likely to have some colleagues at earlier stages, and how you can work with them while also moving the change forward can be a difficult balancing act.

At this point people need to feel that things are going reasonably well, and, perhaps even more importantly, that if problems occur they are dealt with, that concerns are listened to, acted upon, that everyone is kept informed of what is happening, and that progress is reported on (Bacall, 2000; Reed and Turner,

2005). Things may not go to plan and you may need to move to a backup plan or sidestep a problem. If things seem not to be working out, it is worth stopping to look at exactly what is going wrong or differently from how you planned before assuming everything is failing and giving up (unless that is necessary to maintain safety). Recalling your ultimate aim and deciding whether this setback really takes you off track, or whether it is a delay or detour that you can accommodate, and still ultimately get to the same place, is important.

Prochanska and DiClemente's (1992) fifth or final stage of change is that of maintaining change. Unless the change is sustained (provided of course that there is not a good reason why it should be dropped), then the effort devoted to implementing it is time which you could have used on something else. Despite being the last, this can be the most challenging stage. Even when effecting change is difficult, your attention and energy and that of your supporters are on the project. As time goes on, other priorities come along and it is easy to take your eye off the ball (Balasubramanian *et al.*, 2010). Until the change in practice is the new norm, or complete 'refreezing' for everyone in Lewin's (1951) terms has occurred, those who have never come on board can still convince your supporters to go back to how things were, and a constant drip feed of discouragement may mean that the project ultimately fails even after apparent success. It is therefore useful at the planning stage to identify how a new way of working will be maintained. This may include making sure that the equipment and supplies needed to sustain change are always available, and publicizing successes (Golden, 2006). Many changes could also herald further practice development, and it can be useful to start setting the next goal, to keep the enthusiasts on board and to give a clear message that this change is here to stay.

Motivating managers to allow changed practice

Management support for any change is important (Bacall, 2000) and it will usually be appropriate for your manager to at least be aware of the changes which are being made in their department. In many cases you may absolutely require not just permission, but support from your manager. The change you are proposing may require resources in terms of funding, time, or facilities, which will necessitate managerial approval. Managerial support may be necessary in order to reduce the anxieties which your peers have about any adverse effects of change, such as complaints being made or the legal implications of moving to new practice. Your manager is also likely to know what other changes are planned and how these may affect your project. They may be well placed to support your position to more senior management or members of other professions, and to help and encourage you to publicize success. It is always useful when you are initiating change to have someone who is able to provide you with support if the going gets tough, and although your manager may not always be the right person to do this, having them on board may open up an extra avenue of support.

Gaining managerial support may involve assessing whether whoever has to officially approve your idea is at a stage when they are ready for this change.

If your managers are keen for your project to go ahead, then so much the better, but you may need to convince them that it is important. The way in which you seek to achieve this may be different from how you seek to convince colleagues, because the issues that most concern them may be different. You may well feel that what you propose will enhance patient care and that this should be enough. That would be nice. However, there are many ways in which patient care could be enhanced, and budget holders and managers often have multiple demands on their resources and need to know that any expenditure, be it direct costs, time taken to change practice, or a risk of staff becoming disgruntled, will be balanced by the potential for positive outcomes. It is useful to be clear about the possible range of both short and long term benefits, for example in terms of patient outcomes, patient satisfaction, safety, increased efficiency or reduced resource utilization, improved long term staff satisfaction or staff retention which your idea may bring with it. There are usually a number of forces driving organizations, and targets which must be met. If your project will contribute to, feed into, or at least not detract from these, it may be more attractive than just of itself.

As far as possible, it is a good idea to have a fairly clear but flexible plan of how you intend to orchestrate the proposed change when you discuss your ideas with your manager. If time and resources are being considered, then they will want to know that it is well thought out plan and worth investing in. It may also be useful to have some idea of whether the staff who will be required to enact the change support you, because the resources, effort and time which will be required to bring people on board may be an important consideration. How 'ready' you feel your colleagues are for change may also affect when any financial support or other resources which you require will be needed.

You may find that your manager wants to be very involved in your project, and the temptation is often to enthusiastically welcome them. This can be very useful, but it may also be important from the point of view of keeping frontline col leagues on board that the project is clearly owned at workforce level and not seen as part of a management agenda. You may have to tread tactfully and carefully in winning support, making the right concessions and getting the right involvement from each level of staff without alienating others, or losing the focus of your project. Only you can make that decision, and it may not be an easy one.

Changing multidisciplinary practice

Healthcare almost always occurs in situations where disciplines work closely together, and often a change instigated by one group of professionals impacts on or requires the involvement, approval, or co-operation of one or more other professions. For some changes to occur, more than one profession has to agree to change their practice. In others, it may be that one profession is primarily affected but others are indirectly affected, for example because the availability of another profession changes. Sometimes there may be no direct impact for a particular profession, but it can be useful for all team members to know about what their colleagues are doing and to share ideas. In some situations there may be no reason for involving more than one profession except that an individual or group feels that they should be involved and informed, and doing so will make life easier all round.

When a number of professional groups need to be involved in a change in practice, being very clear about how and why each group should be involved is helpful in planning the change process. While wide consultation and involvement has many benefits, there is also a need for clarity over who actually needs to be involved, to what level, and to what end (Scott *et al.*, 2003). This may include deciding whose opinions are being sought to influence a decision, who are simply being informed of a change in practice, whether all groups will hold equal weighting in planning and effecting change, or whether one or two should dominate (Scott *et al.*, 2003). The reasons for your decisions will usually concern whom the change in practice will have the greatest effect on, and whose ownership of it is essential. You may be introducing a new way of administering intravenous drugs and will need to decide whether medical staff need to be involved because they will also administer the drugs, because they prescribe them and thus have some interest in how the drugs are given, because you feel they may have some useful knowledge to contribute, or because the consultants feel they should know. The answer to this is likely to influence what type of involvement medical staff should have, how you manage that, the weighting which is given to their views, and which members of medical staff you involve.

When you are dealing with change that involves the multi disciplinary team you are likely to need to gauge the readiness for change of nurses, physiotherapists, medical staff, dieticians, occupational therapists, and others, and plan change which takes into account the concerns and enthusiasms of all these groups, as well as the individuals within them (Saull-McCaig *et al.*, 2006). In addition to determining whether individuals within professional groups are ready for change, whether professions as a whole are ready for change matters: for example whether there are any issues related to professional ethos which might affect or be affected by the change, whether a particular profession has recently undergone any other significant change, and what additional pressures are currently being applied to each profession. While physiotherapists might individually and as a group, in principle, support a change in practice suggested by the occupational therapy team, they might also be under pressure to achieve other targets which are specific to their own profession, and to which they need to devote the majority of their time and energies.

Working in a multi disciplinary context will probably mean that you need to identify and make use of change agents and opinion leaders across professions. Finding people who will support and work with you in different professions and who will take responsibility within their group can make things much more manageable, as well as securing ownership across professions (Saull-McCaig *et al.*, 2006). They may know the relationships between staff within that profession, and whose opinion really counts. They are also more likely to be seen by their colleagues as understanding and empathizing with them. It can also, however, be necessary to take into account the relationships between individuals across different professions. You may find that the most influential person for the medical consultant is a healthcare assistant whom they consider to be well informed on the day to day practicalities of the ward, and what will and will not work, not the ward manager or the registrars. You may find that bringing the head physiotherapist on board means that the respiratory consultant will automatically veto your idea. Multidisciplinary change management is not easy, and as well as trying to gauge who will influence whom within and across professions, keeping a clear vision of what your goals are can help you to make focused decisions about whom to involve, how to involve people and what agendas from various professions you can take on board or absorb without losing sight of your goal.

Summary

Changing team practice is likely to be much more complex than changing your own practice. However, the same basic processes apply. It involves deciding exactly what you want to change, how you will go about it, identifying things that will help or hinder your plans, how ready people are for change, who the key players are, where they stand in relation to your proposed change, how multidisciplinary team members will be involved, how your managers will be involved and how you will sustain new practice.

Finally, having done all that, you need to decide whether or not the change in practice has happened and been effective, by evaluating it.

Evaluating new practice

12

This chapter discusses what might be considered the final stage of using research in practice: evaluating any changes which have been made because of research findings.

Evaluating changed practice is just as important as all the preceding stages, because you need to know if a new way of doing things works, and creates some sort of improvement (Cork, 2005). Even if you think that it will be obvious whether something works or not, having evidence of this can be useful for addressing criticisms, seeking ongoing support or gaining permission to abandon something which is not working. It can also sometimes highlight areas where you could make things even better than they are, or, if you think all is doom and gloom, you may be surprised to find that things are not quite as bad as you think (Pryjmachuk, 1996; Skinner, 2004).

Evaluation should be the natural continuation of the rest of the process of change (Skinner, 2004). To implement change effectively you need to know exactly what it is that you are aiming to change, and to evaluate changed practice you need to know what you expected to happen, and how you will know whether this has happened or not.

What should be evaluated?

Evaluation of new practice should ideally give a comprehensive picture of what has happened because of the changes made. It should firstly tell you whether what you think is happening or what was meant to happen really is. If you have introduced multidisciplinary documentation, everyone may claim that they use it, but unless you find out whether they actually do, you will have no idea about whether a change in practice has occurred. If you do not know whether people are filling out the new documentation, then you have no way of finding out whether it has had a positive effect or not.

Secondly, evaluation should be designed to tell you if the change in practice is having a positive effect. It is all very well to know that everyone is filling in the multidisciplinary notes but it is also important to know if these improve patient care, efficiency, or multidisciplinary communication. If all they do is create chaos and detract from patient care, then even if everyone is diligently complying, things have not improved, and may even have got worse.

Finally, to be really useful, the evaluation has to be able to ask why something is happening or not, or works or does not (Blamey and MacKenzie, 2007). You may discover that the new multidisciplinary notes which everyone had agreed to use are not being completed, but to decide what the next step is, you need to know why they are not being completed. It may be that the idea is good but quite impractical, or that there is something specific and alterable that is stopping this from happening. Equally if the new notes are being used but causing chaos, then you need to know why this is, so that you can decide whether to make adjustments and try again, or abandon the whole thing.

The sequence of evaluation is important. The first thing you need to know is whether something is happening or not. If you evaluate whether a new approach to documentation has improved multidisciplinary communication on the assumption that it is happening, find a negative effect, and assume that the new documentation has caused it, your assumption may be flawed. You may later discover that the change in practice had never occurred and you were evaluating the effect of nothing.

When to evaluate?

If the change you are implementing has several stages, you should probably aim to do some form of evaluation at every point: there is no point in moving to stage two of your plan if you are not sure if stage one has happened, particularly if stage two depends on stage one having been completed successfully. Some of these evaluations will probably be fairly simple. The first part of your plan for introducing new documentation might be to present the proposed paperwork to all those who will be affected by it, over a one-month period, and to invite feedback on your plans. It would be useful to evaluate whether the majority of staff have heard about your ideas and had the opportunity to comment before moving on to stage two of tweaking the documentation in accordance with feedback, and piloting it. The evaluation at this stage might simply be a list of all the staff with a tick against those whom you have met with. This should reduce the problem of not enough people knowing about the new documentation at the point when you want to pilot it, and individuals giving you their views on whether the tool looks good in principle when you have made a prototype and rolled out the pilot. It may also be useful at this stage to investigate any whys. If you arranged several meetings but found that you were struggling to get everyone to attend, it might be useful to ask why this is. Low attendance could signal a lack of enthusiasm, or poor staffing levels, which could both be problematic when you try to implement new practice.

The final stage of implementing new practice is often where the most comprehensive evaluation needs to be, because this is where you have introduced the change in practice in its entirety and want to know if it works. The evaluation should be focused on exactly what you want to know about the new way of doing things. If you have introduced multidisciplinary documentation, you will probably want to evaluate whether or not it is used, but you also need to be clear about what you mean by 'used': you may want to evaluate whether it is used at all, whether it is used as it should be, and whether all the professions involved use it equally well. That all pertains to whether or not the new documentation is used. It would also be useful to look at the 'whys': for example, why it is not being used as planned, or why certain professions are markedly different from others in their use of it. Whether the new documentation has a positive influence on practice is also important. The ideal might perhaps be to know whether or not it improves care, but it might be impossible to really measure that without carrying out quite a complex piece of evaluation which takes into account all kinds of variables. You might nonetheless be able to get an overview of whether it seems to have had any positive effect by asking staff from various disciplines what they think of the new approach to documentation.

Approaches to evaluation

The right way to evaluate new practice depends on what you are evaluating. As Chapter 2 identified, there are a lot of similarities between the processes followed in research and evaluation, and the question that arises in research, about whether to use qualitative, quantitative or a combination of approaches to getting information also applies when you are deciding how to evaluate new practice (Skinner, 2004). To make this decision, you need to look at the aim(s) or objective(s) which you are evaluating, the nature of these, and decide what sort of information you need in order to evaluate them. If you are evaluating an aim which would be best assessed using numerical measurement, then your evaluation should use methods of gathering information which will achieve this. If what you need to know is more about personal experiences, views, attitudes or values, then you probably need to use 'qualitative' approaches (Reid *et al.*, 2007).

If you are evaluating how many staff have attended meetings about new documentation, you will almost certainly use numerical scores. If you find that very few have attended and want to find out why, then you will probably want to talk to those who have not attended. This may be best achieved using a qualitative approach, especially if you want to find out the real reason why they did not attend, rather than just that they were 'too busy' (they probably were, but you want to know why your project was low priority). So, even a fairly simple evaluation point may require two methods of collecting data. If you have an action plan with several points which you will evaluate, then it is very likely that the plan as a whole will require a mix of approaches to evaluation. Essentially, though, the way you seek information should be guided by what type of information you are looking for.

Evaluation methods

There are no right or wrong evaluation methods: it depends on what you are evaluating. You might use questionnaires, observation, analysis of documents, interviews (with individuals or groups), pre and post tests, and many more. Whichever tool or tools you use need to be designed to assess, measure or investigate exactly what you want to know about (Reid *et al.*, 2007). If you want to check whether or not new documentation is completed, then you might decide to use documentary evidence: look and see if the notes are completed using the new paperwork. If you also want to know what the staff think of this approach to documentation, you might use questionnaires, or hold individual or group interviews with staff to ascertain their views.

You may need to use more than one method of evaluation in order to get the whole picture of how a new approach is working, or to detect any differences between rhetoric, intentions, beliefs and what actually happens in practice (Haveri, 2008). For example, you may use discussions or questionnaires to find out what the staff think, or say they think, of the new documentation, and document analysis to see what happens in practice.

Even if the evaluation you are planning seems fairly straightforward, it can be useful to think through exactly what you need to find out, and how you can match what you would ideally like to know with what you have the time to achieve. If you are going to evaluate whether or not a new approach to documentation is used, you may decide that you want to numerically measure, over a one-week period, whether or not the new documents are used. That may mean that you will need a tick-box evaluation tool of how many recordings are made, where and by which professional groups. You will also have to decide on the sample you need: whether you will take all the notes everyday and check them, or use a sample that you think is a reasonable representation, and check those. To make this decision you would need to think about how many sets of notes each option means there will be, where they will be (for instance, whether you will have to go to other wards and departments to gather them), how much time it will take, and if you will have the time available for it. You may have to opt for something less than perfect but manageable.

You also need to decide on exactly what you want to measure: for example, whether you just want to know how many notes were completed using the new documentation and how many still used the old system, or whether you want a means of documenting when the notes in question were completed (so that you can trace things like whether it being night or day or the weekend seemed to have any influence), which professional groups were involved and what grade within the profession made the notes. Although you need to consider every point which might require evaluation, there is also benefit in not making the potentially simple complex unless you have to. Before you get too involved in deciding how to find the time and facilities to sit and cross check records against time, staff group and grade, it might be worth starting with a simple evaluation of whether or not the new documentation was used. If 100 per cent of the notes were recorded using the new system, then you do not need to worry about the complexity of when and by whom. It can be worth getting the overall picture before worrying too much about the minutiae, because you may not need to.

Sometimes a change in practice brings outcomes (good and bad) which were not expected, and which have therefore not been catered for in the official evaluation strategy (Reed and Turner, 2005). Because you will not know what the evaluation will show, you need to keep an open mind about the possibility to changing or adding to your approach to evaluation as you go, so your methods should not be set in stone. Evaluation of new practice also occurs in the real world, where all kinds of things happen which are nothing to do with whatever you are evaluating. You will nearly always have to think about distinguishing what happens because of a change in practice from things which happen at about the same time and might look related, but are not actually anything to do with the new practice. This might include staffing levels, organizational change outside your project, competing priorities and a whole host of other things (Blamey and Makenzie, 2007). This makes the why questions very important and, although careful planning is important, you have to be prepared to go off your original script. You may have planned to measure over a two-week period how often the new documentation is used and how often people use the old documents, noting also which professional group makes each entry. In addition, you may have planned as your 'why' part of the evaluation to hold three group discussions on people's views on the new documentation with a range of staff from across professional groups. If the first part of the evaluation shows that 80 per cent of entries in the notes now use the new documentation, but the 20 per cent that do not are all occupational therapy notes, you might change your plans. Instead of holding three group discussions with a range of staff members, you might decide to explore if there is an issue for occupational therapists by holding a meeting with them. You might find from this that the occupational therapy team currently have two people on long-term sick leave, and are relying heavily on bank staff who do not know about the new documents. The fact that the occupational therapy team appear not to be participating is nothing to do with the new documentation or occupational therapists' views of it, it is about their staffing situation at present.

Because you are evaluating real-world events, probably in your own workplace, you are also likely to have the option of unplanned evaluation opportunities. These are often very valuable and the fact that they are not a part of your planned evaluation strategy does not mean that you should ignore them. If you overhear two colleagues talking about a small group of staff who refuse to use the new documentation, then you may have a very useful lead as to people whom you need to meet with in order to find out what they oppose about the new system. It would be foolish to decide that because your evaluation strategy does not include hanging around the sluice listening to other people's conversations you cannot act on this. You may not want to dig out the members of staff concerned, name the colleagues who were talking about them and repeat what they said, but you might well use this information to decide who to talk to or invite to discussion groups.

Who or what to collect information from?

Sometimes where or from whom you should collect data is quite obvious. If you are evaluating whether or not new multidisciplinary documentation is completed, then the multidisciplinary notes are the most obvious choice of place to get the information. However, it may not always be that easy. If you decide to ask staff their views on the new system of documentation, you need to decide whether you want data from everyone, from all staff groups, from a particular staff group or particular individuals. You should try to be very clear on who you need to ask and why. This includes thinking about how you choose the people to ask: if you ask for volunteers to attend a discussion about the new documentation, the chances are you will get those who like it and want to say so, and those who want to complain, but few people who are 'middle of the road'. If you specifically invite a selection of people, you may be more likely to get a variety of views and may be able to aim for a better mix of staff groups than asking for volunteers might achieve. However, it may mean that people who have a particularly interesting opinion which they wish to share are inadvertently excluded. Your job as the person designing the evaluation is to choose the best sample for the job: the one that will get the most accurate information, while also being achievable.

Who should gather data?

It is important to think about who will gather the information that you need. Your decisions are likely to be driven in part by feasibility, but also by what effect different individuals gathering the data may have on it. The ideal might be for you to gather all the data yourself. However, if this is not a realistic task for one person, you will need to enlist assistance. If more than one person is collecting the information, then you need to be sure that everyone is evaluating as close as possible to the same thing. This may be relatively easy if you are just recording whether or not documents are used, but it may sometimes be necessary to be very clear about what is being evaluated, and how the evaluation is being conducted.

Another issue to consider is whether the person collecting the information will affect what people say or do. If you want to find out why a group of staff are not completing the documentation that you have just introduced, they may not answer truthfully if you are collecting the data. They may not want to hurt your feelings, they may feel unable to criticize your project to your face, and if they are deliberately trying to sabotage the project you will probably not get an honest answer. It may also be difficult for you to ask people in a completely unbiased manner why they are not supporting your project. So it can be worth getting someone else to gather that information. Conversely you may not feel convinced that another person really knows enough about the project to hold the evaluation conversations, so despite the possible limitations, you may be the most ideal data collector.

The role and position of anyone who is assisting you to collect evaluation data merit consideration. If a manager is collecting the information, staff may fear that it is being gathered to monitor their performance, rather than to evaluate the new way of doing things. As well as the position and role of the person collecting the information, it is important to think about the skills and attributes of the person or people who assist you. If you are trying to gather and record data in a logical and organized way, then a person who is known to be disorganized and to struggle with recording things diligently may not be your ideal person for the task, even if they are very enthusiastic. On the other hand, if you want someone to talk to staff, a person who easily gains people's confidence and is good at listening may be the best choice, even if their organizational skills are not of a high order. Practically, you also need someone who has enough time for, and commitment to, the project to do the necessary work.

Biases

When you design your evaluation, you need to think about things that might make your findings biased or inaccurate. This may happen because of design flaws in the evaluation, for example, in the way that you ask questions, observe practice, check documents, etc. and how far what you are assessing in the evaluation addresses your original objectives. You may also want to think about time-related factors that might affect the apparent results of your evaluation. If you are evaluating the use of new multidisciplinary notes, it might not be ideal to carry out your evaluation during the week when the new junior doctors start work, and where errors may be about them getting used to documentation in general, not the new documents per se.

As well as design faults in the evaluation, it may be difficult for you to be unbiased about your project, because you are likely to want it to work. If you have been allowed time and resources to make a change in practice, there may be pressure on you to show that it has worked, is being done or has created improvement of some kind. While this may not mean that you would deliberately spin your evaluation, it does create pressure to show that things are working well. However, you have to be sure that you are setting up an evaluation to see how things are working, not to prove success.

If you are using other people to assist you, you have to consider their possible biases as well as your own: and not just their positive biases. In Chapter 11 the possibility of encouraging people who do not really support a change in practice to join the project team in order to increase their enthusiasm was highlighted. It can be useful to remember this when you are designing the evaluation, and perhaps ensuring that they are not solely responsible for evaluating a part of the project which they never supported in the first place.

When to collect data?

You may need to collect evaluative information on your project at a number of points, but the timing of the final evaluation usually requires more thought than the preceding stages. The interim stages are usually progressive and you know how long each one is meant to last. If you decided to hold information-giving sessions on a regular basis over a four-week period and then evaluate how many people had attended, you know that you will do this after four weeks. In contrast, deciding when to evaluate whether practice has actually changed can be more difficult.

You need time for the change in practice to have happened, and to show an effect, before you evaluate it. If you introduce new documentation, you may want to wait two weeks or so while everyone gets used to it and can ask you about teething problems before you monitor whether or not the new notes are used. If you want to evaluate the effect of new practice, you may need to wait longer than you do to evaluate whether it has happened or not. For example, if you wanted to see whether a new method of documentation was linked with a reduction in re-admissions, you would probably need to leave it a few months at least before you could look at the numbers of readmissions, re-referrals etc to evaluate whether the new approach seemed to have contributed to this.

It is usually a good idea not to rely entirely on the time just after new practice has been introduced to evaluate whether it is happening and whether it works well. As Chapter 11 identified, one problem with introducing new practice can be that it initially works well, but people then lose the enthusiasm to sustain it, other priorities come along, what was working well starts to stumble, and slowly everyone reverts to the old way of doing things (Balasubramanian *et al.*, 2010). To avoid this, it may be useful to plan short-term, medium-term and ongoing evaluations. For example, evaluating whether new documents are used four weeks after they are introduced, six months later or after a year. This can help to sustain your own and other people's interest in the project, and to identify if practice has really changed, and whether the new practice is sustainable.

Interpreting data

Gathering information is all very well, but you need to decide what it means. How you do this depends largely on what type of data you collect.

If you have gathered numerical data, it needs to be dealt with using numerical means. Sometimes how you will interpret the information that you have gathered hardly requires any thought: for instance, if you are checking how many staff have attended information-giving sessions, you count the number and see how many did and did not attend. Although you may be using what seems to be a quantitative approach, as discussed in relation to research in Chapter 5, in many evaluations that involve just one team, ward or unit, you are unlikely to get into any depth of statistical analysis: you are likely to be looking at raw scores, percentages or other descriptive statistics. This is usually completely acceptable, because you are not likely to have a sample size that is large enough to do more, and because you usually just want to see if the change in practice works in the environment you want to use it in. If you are carrying out a larger-scale evaluation or an evaluation from which you intend to claim wide generalizations, then you need to think about using inferential statistics (see Chapter 5). However, you only need to do this if the scale or intention of your evaluation merits it.

You may sometimes not only need to decide how to numerically analyse information, but to decide what level of achievement is acceptable. If you are looking for how many people are completing multidisciplinary notes, you need to decide how many an acceptable level is. If you find that 100 per cent of staff are using the new notes, then that of course is fine, but unless things are that good, you need to decide what level makes it seem worth carrying on without much further intervention, what level means that more input is needed and what level means a major rethink.

If your data is qualitative, then your way of analysing it needs to match this, for example, as described in the context of research in Chapter 6, by looking at the information which you have and coding and categorizing it or arranging it into themes. If you are collecting more than one type of data, you need to think, as Chapter 7 described, about how you will tie it all together, for instance, how you will link scores related to whether documents were used or not with the codes developed from the qualitative analysis.

Ethics and evaluation

If you are carrying out an evaluation, you have obligations to those participating in the evaluation; the ward, team or unit involved; and the organization as a whole (Hughes, 2008). The requirements to provide benefit, respect autonomy seek justice and do no harm apply equally to conducting evaluation of new practice as to every other aspect of healthcare provision. Usually, an evaluation of changed practice will not require approval by an ethics committee. It is more likely that the change in practice as a whole, including the evaluation strategy, will have required approval through local governance processes.

The obligation to do no harm and to do good is often used as a reason why evaluation of new practice should take place. Some might argue that introducing new practice without investigating whether this has any positive outcomes is unethical, as you have no idea of the effect which it has on individual patients, groups of patients, publicly funded resources, etc. unless you evaluate it. Whereas in research the question is, 'is it ethical to conduct the research, in evaluation of new practice'? The question may rather be whether it would be ethical not to evaluate it.

The requirement for evaluation to be conducted ethically is as high as the requirement for research to be conducted ethically (Wade, 2005). In terms of doing good and doing no harm, if practice has changed, and the new way of doing things will continue unless there is evidence that it should not, the need for evaluation to be accurate and honest is very high, because it is almost certain that patient care, staff or other resources will be affected by it.

The principle of respect for autonomy applies to evaluation in a similar way that it does to research. You may be gathering data which relates to individuals or groups, and whether these individuals have consented to this (and whether they need to) has to be considered. In some cases consent may not be an issue: if you were collecting information about whether new documentation was completed accurately over a one-week period of time, then you probably would not need to gain consent from all the patients involved to look at their notes, unless you were also noting their names. On the other hand, if a part of your evaluation was to talk with patients to explore their views on whether staff seemed to know what each other were doing or had done, or if you were collecting data from colleagues, you would need to give them enough information to provide informed consent or decline to participate. You would also need to consider issues surrounding coercion to participate, fear of reprisals for non-participation or for what was said, confidentiality of information and how this information was stored, shared and used. You might only wish to know about a colleague's views to evaluate your project, but they could fear that their views would be identifiable by managers and used in evidence against them in other contexts.

Sharing the findings

It is likely that a variety of people will have invested in some way in the change you have implemented, and you have an obligation to let them know the outcome of their efforts. The way in which you do this depends in part on the nature and scope of the change concerned. It may be that you have the backing of the organization you work for as a whole, your manager and have sought the support of your immediate colleagues. In this case, you may need to write a report for your manager and/or employer, and also think of meaningful ways to let your colleagues know what the outcomes of the new way of working are. This might be through meetings, a project report or a poster in the ward or department. Everyone who has given time and commitment should be able to know the outcome of their work, firstly out of courtesy, but also because unless people know what is happening because of their efforts there is no reason for them to continue to co-operate, or to assist you with future endeavours (Pryjmachuk, 1996; Skinner, 2004).

Planning ongoing change

Evaluation is often seen as the last stage of change, and you might feel it would be nice if it was. By this stage you may feel like taking a well-earned vacation. However, having conducted the evaluation of new practice, you then need to decide what to do because of it. You may find that the new way of working is effective and has remained so for a year, so you can sit back and relax for a bit.

However, you may have to decide whether to encourage people to continue with the new way of doing things or not. Sometimes there is obvious benefit, everyone is doing as planned and there is no decision to make. In other cases the results are not so clear cut. You may need to decide whether to put in the time and effort to bring more people on board, and whether to change some aspect of the new way of working to try to achieve this. The new way of doing things may have brought some improvement but also some problems, and you may need to decide whether the benefits outweigh the costs, and the direction which ongoing practice should take.

Even when things have gone to plan, everything is going well, your colleagues are enthusiastic and patients are delighted, your work may not be done. There may now be a logical next step which you need to take. If you have introduced multidisciplinary documentation for discharge planning, and it has been a huge success, you may feel obliged, or even be obliged, to think about working on more general multidisciplinary notes. Don't you just hate it when doing a good job gives you more work?

Summary

If new practice has been introduced, it should really be evaluated, so that you know whether it works or not, if anyone has benefited, and whether it is worth continuing with. This includes looking at whether there has really been a change in practice, whether the expected benefits have materialized, whether the new way of doing things has created any problems, and thinking about unexpected outcomes as well as the expected effects. It is also important to look at the reasons for the outcomes, so that you know whether or not they were really linked to the new way of working, or just a coincidence.

Any evaluation should be logically and systematically designed, so that nothing is missed or assumed, and the way in which information is gathered and analysed should be appropriate to the matter in question. If possible, it is useful to evaluate new ways of working in the short, medium and long term, so that you get an idea of the benefits and challenges over time, as well as in the immediate aftermath of the effort devoted to changing practice. It is also important to give feedback to those who have supported you, have been involved in, or will be affected by, the new way of working.

Conclusion

Hopefully the language which is used in research is now clearer, finding information may be less arduous and what you should evaluate in a research report is manageable. There are few perfect studies, and your task is not so much to see if a study was perfect but to decide whether it was good enough to pay any attention to, how much attention to give it, how much weight it should have compared to the rest of the evidence, and, perhaps most vitally, how you can use it in practice.

Changing your own practice, and persuading others to change theirs, is probably a much harder task than understanding and evaluating research, and requires a good deal of thought, planning and sometimes determination. The scale of your plans will depend on how many people and services are involved, but it is useful to think about everything that might stand in the way of even the most apparently straightforward change in practice, how you can set things up to overcome or avoid the problems and who and what will help things to run as smoothly as possible. Once a new way of working has been set up, it is important to check whether it works and benefits anyone. The process of finding this out should be systematic and logical, and enable you to decide whether it is worth continuing with.

It is also useful to be realistic about what you can do: it is unlikely that you can check the evidence for every aspect of practice in your area of work, and do something about everything that could be improved. The most that the majority of us can do is to identify one area of practice that we can and want to look at, and then focus on that. Doing that is better than being so paralysed by the enormity of the task of changing the world that nothing happens. If you find and evaluate the research about one aspect of practice, and make, or take a part in making, one change to improve things, one thing improves. If you do nothing, you don't need me to tell you what has changed.

If you have developed a new way of doing things, it is useful to let others know about this. There may be some people that you have to let know, because they provided resources for, or allowed, the project, because you have to report to them about what you get up to, or because they were involved in or will be affected by the new way of working. However, there are also likely to be people outside your obligatory and good manners reporting circle who would find your experience useful to know.

This may not be what you want to hear, and I hate to leave on a bad note, but it can be very useful if ways of using evidence in practice are made public knowledge. You might feel that unless you have done a really top-class piece of research, you do not have anything to publicize. The reality is the opposite. It is all very well to have a really good piece of research, but unless people know how it could work in practice, it often stays on the shelf and has no impact at all. So, a report on how evidence has been used in practice can be the most useful type of publication.

When people talk about publicizing what you have done, it can create a spectre of being expected to sit down and write something lengthy and academic when there are more interesting things on offer. Of course, if you want to do that, there is no reason not to, but it is not essential for getting evidence into the public domain. Part of how you decide to disseminate information is personal preference. Some people enjoy conferences: they are a great way of sharing information, and usually have different presentation options; so you can put in for a small group presentation or poster if you feel that a large main hall event is not what you want to do, or what suits what you have to say. Another option is journals, and there are such a range of them that there is bound to be at least one that will be suitable for what you have been involved in. A lot of journals have different sections, some of which report research, and others which report innovations in practice, evaluations of practice or case studies of good practice; so there is very likely to be a suitable slot for you to publicize your evidence and share your experiences.

If all this sounds a bit too formal, there are plenty of both online and face-to-face special-interest groups which may like to hear about what you have done, and it may be worth asking if your work can be presented in some way on the staff intranet, or the organization's newsletter. Your organization may also have a way of posting examples of good practice on their website: that way, anyone who 'Googles' can find out what you did and what worked. That is why the Internet can be very useful for grey literature.

For the whole evidence-based practice to work, the people who are holding the most important part of the jigsaw puzzle are the people who have changed, or attempted to change, practice, however small a part of it, and who know what works and what does not, and why. If you have the best bit of the puzzle, you may need to keep it to the end so that you know exactly where it goes, but after you have let everyone else scrabble around looking for it for a while, please put it in!

Appendix 1: Deciding whether to use a study's findings

The following questions may be a useful reminder of what to look for in a piece of research.

What is the study about?
- Title
- Hypothesis/question/problem statement/statement of intent

Background
- Is there a literature review?
- Does the literature review seem to be thorough, unbiased and relevant to the study?

Paradigm, design and methodology
- Are these stated?
- Do they seem to fit the subject?
- Do the paradigm, design and methodology match each other?

Methods
- Do these seem to be a sensible way of finding out the information required?
- Does the way they were used match the methodology/paradigm?
- Does anything about them seem likely to produce misleading results?
- Were any procedures or tools that were used developed appropriately (e.g., piloted, discussed with a panel of experts)?

Sample
- Was the way the sample was selected appropriate for this study?
- Are the samples taken from the population that the study was meant to be about?

- Would the way in which the sample was selected place any limitations on the results?
- Was the sample an appropriate size for the type of research?
- Was the response rate high enough (if relevant?)

Ethical issues

Were these considered?
For example:

- ethics review
- informed consent
- potential harm
- any evidence of coercion to participate
- confidentiality and anonymity

Data analysis

- Was the right approach used? (e.g., qualitative analysis for qualitative data)
- Were appropriate specific analysis procedures used? (e.g., statistical tests)

For quantitative research

- Were descriptive or inferential statistics used, and was this appropriate?
- Were parametric or non-parametric tests used and was this appropriate?
- Were appropriate specific statistical tests used?
- Were the power, p value and confidence interval and level commented on if inferential statistics were used?

For qualitative research

- Were all the data sources analysed?
- Were the data analysis strategies clearly described?
- Was there evidence that codes/themes/categories were developed logically and within the ethos of the study?
- Is there enough evidence (e.g., quotes used) to support the findings?
- Was enough contextual information provided for you to consider the transferability of the study?

Reliability and validity/trustworthiness

- Does it appear that the study was conducted systematically?
- Was anything obvious missing?
- Was there anything that might have meant that the results could be misleading, or due to something other than what was being investigated?

For quantitative research

- Were reliability, internal validity in terms of construct validity, content validity, criterion validity (where appropriate) and external validity addressed?
- Were all the data accounted for (no missing results)?

For qualitative research

- Were the steps the researcher took to ensure the 'truth' of their findings clear?
- Consider evaluating trustworthiness in terms of credibility, transferability and dependability.

For mixed methods research

- Were the data analysis processes appropriate for the type of data in question, and was there evidence of appropriate integration of results?

What were the results/findings?

- Do these make sense?
- Are they clearly related to the study hypothesis/question/problem statement/statement of intent?
- Are the results consistent with the methodology, methods and sampling?
- Are any other things which might have influenced the results accounted for?
- If mixed methods were used, are the findings appropriately integrated?

Are there clear conclusions and recommendations?

- Do the conclusions and recommendations match the findings?
- Are the conclusions presented with the appropriate degree of certainty given the methodology, study design and findings?

Appendix 2: Was an appropriate statistical test used?

These are some of the commonly used statistical tests, and the type of decision trail which can guide you about whether or not the right tests were used (Motulsky, 1995).

Other tests and combinations of tests also exist.

A2.1 Are the data parametric or non-parametric?

Parametric data	Non-parametric data
Descriptive statistics Mean Standard Deviation	**Descriptive statistics** Median, Mode, Percentage
Inferential statistics Compare 1 group with a hypothetical variable: 1 sample t test	**Inferential statistics** Compare 1 group with a hypothetical variable: Wilcoxon's test　　　　　Chi Square
Compare 2 groups: t-test (paired or unpaired dependant on whether groups were paired)	Compare two groups (unmatched): Mann-Whitney U Test　　Chi square, Fisher's
	Compare two groups (matched): Wilcoxon's Test　　　　　McNemar's
To compare more than 2 groups: ANOVA	Compare more than 2 groups: Friedman (matched groups)　　Chi square Kruskal-Wallis(unmatched groups)

Appendix 3: Action plan template examples

A3.1 Project aim:

Objectives	Actions required	People involved	Resources needed	Review date	Evaluation criteria

A3.2 Goal:

Objective	How this will be achieved and by whom	Resources needed	How achievement of the objective will be evaluated	Target date

Appendix 4: Additional resources

Books

Andrews, S. and Halcomb, E. J. 2009. *Mixed Methods Research for Nursing and the Health Sciences.* Chichester: Wiley-Blackwell Publishing.
This book provides a practical guide to designing, conducting and reporting mixed methods research in nursing and the health sciences.

Cutliffe, J. and Ward, M. 2007. *Critiquing Nursing Research.* London: Quay Books.
This book focuses specifically on critiquing, rather than conducting, nursing research.

Greenhalgh, T. 2010. *How to Read a Paper: The Basics of Evidence-Based Medicine*, 4th edn. Chichester: Wiley-Blackwell.
This book focuses on the principles of evidence-based medicine, and how to critically evaluate a range of types of research paper.

LoBiondo-Wood, G. and Haber, J. 2009. *Nursing Research: Methods and Critical Appraisal for Evidence-Based Practice*, 7th edn. Philadelphia, St Louis and New York: Mosby.
This book provides an introduction to the concepts which underpin nursing research, and the methods of conducting research, including guidance on evaluating studies and applying them to practice.

Polit, D. F. and Beck, C. T. 2009. *Essentials of Nursing Research: Methods, Appraisal, and Utilization.* Philadelphia: Lippincott, Williams and Wilkins.
This book focuses on how to read and evaluate research in order to use it in practice.

Polit, D. F. and Beck, C. T. 2011. *Nursing Research: Generating and Assessing Evidence for Nursing Practice.* 9th revised international edn. Philadelphia: Lippincott Williams & Wilkins.
This book discusses both conducting and critiquing research, and has a strong focus on the link between research and evidence-based practice. It includes a range of tools which can be used to evaluate evidence.

Polit, D. F. and Beck, C. T. 2009. *Study Guide for Essentials of Nursing Research: Appraising Evidence for Nursing Practice.* Philadelphia: Lippincott, Williams and Wilkins.

This guide is designed to accompany *Essentials of Nursing Research* (see above) and provides review exercises related to the topics covered in the textbook.

Web-based resources

(All accessed on 13 January 2011.)
AGREE (http://www.agreecollaboration.org/)
AGREE is an international collaboration of researchers and policymakers who have established a framework for the development, reporting and assessment of clinical practice guidelines.

Centre for Evidence-Based Medicine (http://www.cebm.net)
The website for the centre for evidence based medicine (Oxford) has many sections, including tools and downloads to assist in the critical appraisal of medical evidence.

Cochrane Collaboration (http://www.cochrane.org)
The Cochrane Collaboration website includes the Cochrane library of systematic reviews

Critical Appraisal Skills Programme (http://www.sph.nhs.uk/what-we-do/public-health-workforce/resources/critical-appraisals-skills-programme)
The Critical Appraisal Skills Programme (CASP) aims to enable individuals to develop the skills to find and make sense of research and to use evidence in practice. Their webpages include the Critical Appraisal Skills Programme Tools for evaluating various forms of research.

Health Scotland (http://www.wellscotland.info/evidence/resources/index.aspx)
These pages present five guides related to the evaluation of mental health improvement initiatives.

Involve (http://www.invo.org.uk/)
Involve is an advisory group which supports greater public involvement in British National Health Service, public health and social care research.

Joanna Briggs Institute (http://www.joannabriggs.edu.au/about/home.php)
The Joanna Briggs Institute is an international collaboration involving nursing, medical and allied health researchers, clinicians, academics and quality managers. The website includes a best practice database and library of systematic reviews.

Scottish Intercollegiate Guidelines Network (SIGN) (http://www.sign.ac.uk/)
SIGN develops clinical practice guidelines for the National Health Service (NHS) in Scotland.

'What is' series (http://www.whatisseries.co.uk/whatis/)
The 'What is' series is aimed at demystifying some of the terminology, techniques and practices that are used in research and evidence based practice.

References

Abbott, P. and Sapsford, R. 1998. *Research Methods for Nurses and the Caring Professions (Social Science for Nurses & the Caring Professions)* 2nd edn. Buckingham: Open University Press.

Aleem, I. S., Jalal, H., Aleem, I. S., Sheikh, A. A. and Bhandari, M. 2009. 'Clinical Decision Analysis: Incorporating the Evidence with Patient Preferences', *Patient Preference and Adherence*, 3: 21–4.

Allan, E. 2007. 'Change Management for School Nurses in Scotland', *Nursing Standard* 21,42: 35–9.

Astin, F. 2009. 'A Beginner's Guide to Appraising a Qualitative Research Paper', *British Journal of Cardiac Nursing*, 4,11: 530–3.

Bacall, R. 2000. *The Importance of Leadership in Managing Change*, Ontario: Canada: Bacall and Associates) http://work911.com/articles/leadchange. htm; accessed 2 September 2010.

Balasubramanian, B. A., Chase, S. M., Nutting, P. A., Cohen, D. J., Strickland, P. A., Crosson, J. C., Miller, W. L. and Crabtree, B. F. 2010. 'Using Learning Teams for Reflective Adaptation (ULTRA): Insights From a Team-Based Change Management Strategy in Primary Care', *Annals of Family Medicine*, 8,5: 425–32.

Balls, P. 2009. 'Phenomenology in Nursing Research: Methodology, Interviewing and Transcribing', *Nursing Times*, 105,32–3: 30–3.

Barnett-Page, E. and Thomas, J. 2009. 'Methods for the Synthesis of Qualitative Research: A Critical Review', *BMC Medical Research Methodology*, 9,59, http://www.biomedcentral.com/1471-2288/9/59; accessed 23 November 2009.

Beauchamp, T. L. and Childress, J. F. 2001. *Principles of Biomedical Ethics.* Oxford: Oxford University Press.

Beck, C. T. 2002. 'Postpartum Depression: A Meta Synthesis', *Qualitative Health Research*, 12,4: 453–72.

Benner, P. 1984. *From Novice to Expert: Excellence and Power in Clinical Nursing Practice*. New York, USA: Addison Wesley Publishing.

Bettany-Saltikov, J. 2010. 'Learning How to Undertake a Systematic Review: Part 1', *Nursing Standard*, 24,50: 47–55.

Björkström, M. E. and Hamrin, E. K. F. 2001. 'Swedish Nurses' Attitudes towards Research and Development within Nursing', *Journal of Advanced Nursing*, 34,5: 706–14.

Blaikie, N. 2003. *Analysing Quantitative Data*. London: Sage.

Blamey, A. and Mackenzie, M. 2007. 'Theories of Change and Realistic Evaluation: Peas in a Pod or Apples and Oranges?' *Evaluation*, 13,4: 439–55.

Bonner, A. and Sando, J. 2008. 'Examining the Knowledge, Attitude and Use of Research by Nurses', *Journal of Nursing Management*, 16,3: 334–43.

Bonner, A. and Greenwood, J. 2006. 'The Acquisition and Exercise of Nephrology Nursing Expertise: A Grounded Theory Study', *Journal of Clinical Nursing*, 15,4: 480–9.

Bowles, K. H., Holmes, J. H., Ratcliffe, S. J., Liberatore, M., Nydick, R. and Naylor, M. D. 2009. 'Factors Identified by Experts to Support Decision Making for Post Acute Referral', *Nursing Research*, 58,2:115–22.

Bradley, E. H., Curry, L. A. and Devers, K. J. 2007. 'Qualitative Data Analysis for Health Services Research: Developing Taxonomy, Themes, and Theory', *Health Services Research*, 42,4: 1758–72.

Brenner, M. 2005. 'Children's Nursing in Ireland: Barriers to, and Facilitators of, Research Utilisation', *Paediatric Nursing*, 17,4: 40–5.

Brown, C. and Lloyd, K. 2001. 'Qualitative Methods in Psychiatric Research', *Advances in Psychiatric Treatment*, 7,5: 350–6.

Bryman, A. 2006. 'Integrating Quantitative and Qualitative Research: How is it Done?', *Qualitative Research*, 6,1: 97–113.

Burton, C. 2004. *Understanding How Research is Presented*. London: Distance Learning Centre, South Bank University.

Burck, C. 2005. 'Comparing Qualitative Research Methodologies for Systemic Research: The Use of Grounded Theory, Discourse Analysis and Narrative Analysis', *Journal of Family Therapy*, 27,3: 237–62.

Burla, L. Knierim, B., Barth, J., Liewad, K., Duetz, M. and Abel, T. 2008. 'From Text to Codings', *Nursing Research*, 57,2: 113–17.

Burns, N. and Grove, S. K. 2005. *The Practice of Nursing Research: Conduct, Critique and Utilisation*. 5th edn. Philadelphia USA: WB Saunders.

Bush, H. 2002. 'Inner Strength in Women: Metasynthesis of Qualitative Findings in Theory Development', *Journal of Theory Construction and Testing*, http://www.allbusiness.com/professional-scientific/scientific-research/318659-1.html; accessed 2 September 2010.

Campos, C. J. G. and Turato, E. R. 2009. 'Content Analysis in Studies Using the Clinical-Qualitative Method: Application and Perspectives', *Revista Latino-Americana de Enfermagem*, 17,2: 259–64.

Carrion, M., Woods, P. and Norman, I. 2004. 'Barriers to Research Utilisation among Forensic Mental Health Nurses', *International Journal of Nursing Studies*, 41,6: 613–19.

Carter, S. M. and Little, M. 2007. 'Justifying Knowledge, Justifying Method, Taking Action: Epistemologies, Methodologies, and Methods in Qualitative Examples of Frameworks', *Qualitative Health Research*, 17,10: 1316–28.

Chau, J. P. C., Lopez, V. and Thompson, D. R. 2008. 'A Survey of Hong Kong Nurses' Perceptions of Barriers to, and Facilitators of, Research Utilization', *Research in Nursing and Health*, 31,6: 640–9.

Chin, R. and Benne, K. D. 1985. 'General Strategies for Effecting Change in Human Systems', in W. D. Bennis, K. D. Benne and R. Chin (eds), *The Planning of Change*, 4th edn. New York: Holt Rinehart and Winston, pp. 22–45.

Christensen, M. and Hewitt-Taylor, J. 2006. 'From Expert to Tasks, Expert Nursing Practice Redefined?', *Journal of Clinical Nursing*, 15,12: 1531–9.

Clarke, G. 2001. *Action Planning Hemophilia Organization Development Monograph Series No. 2.* Montreal, Quebec, Canada: World Federation of Hemophilia.

Clifford, C., Murray, S. and Kelly, S. M. 2001. 'A Multiprofessional Perspective of the Role and Training Needs for Research Utilisation in Healthcare', *Journal of Clinical Excellence*, 3,4: 175–82.

Collins, K. M. T., Onwuegbuzie, A. J., and Jiao, Q. G. 2007. 'A Mixed Methods Investigation of Mixed Methods Sampling Designs in Social and Health Science Research', *Journal of Mixed Methods Research*, 1,3: 267–94.

Considine, J., Botti, M. and Thomas, S. 2007. 'Do Knowledge and Experience Have Specific Roles in Triage Decision-Making?' *Academic Emergency Medicine*, 14,8: 722–6.

Cork, A. 2005. 'A Model for Successful Change Management', *Nursing Standard*, 19,25: 40–2.

Coughlan, M., Cronin, P. and Ryan, F. 2007. 'Step by-Step Guide to Critiquing Research. Part 1: Quantitative Research', *British Journal of Nursing*, 16,11: 658–63.

Creswell, J. W. 2003. *Research Design: Qualitative, Quantitative, and Mixed Methods Approaches*, 2nd edn. Thousand Oaks, California, USA: Sage Publications.

Creswell, J. W. and Plano Clark, V. L. 2007. *Designing and Conducting Mixed Methods Research.* Thousand Oaks, California, USA: Sage Publications.

Crombie, I. K. and Davis, H. T. O. 2009. *What is Meta-Analysis?* 2nd edn. Hayward Medical Communications. http://www.whatisseries.co.uk/whatis/pdfs/What_is_meta_analy.pdf; accessed 2 September, 2010.

Curry, L. A., Nembhard, I. M. and Bradley, E. H. 2009 'Qualitative and Mixed Methods Provide Unique Contributions to Outcomes Research', *Circulation*, 119,10:1442–52.

Davies, B., Larson, J., Contro, N., Reyes-Hailey, C., Ablin, A. R., Chesla, C. A., Sourkes, B. and Cohen, H. 2009. 'Conducting a Qualitative Culture Study of Pediatric Palliative Care', *Qualitative Health Research*, 19,1: 5–16.

Deeks, J. J., Higgins, J. P. T. and Altman, D. G. 2009. 'Analysing Data and Undertaking Meta Analyses,' in J. T. P. Higgins and S. Green (eds), *Cochrane Handbook for Systematic Reviews of Interventions, Version 5.0.2.* The Cochrane Collaboration. Available from www.cochrane-handbook.org, accessed 23 July 2010.

Department of Health. 2008. *A High Quality Workforce.* London: Department of Health.

de Jager, P. 2001. 'Resistance to Change: A New View of an Old Problem', *The Futurist*, 35,3: 24–7.

Di Censo, A., Cullum, N. and Ciliska, D. 1998. 'Implementing Evidence-Based Nursing: Some Misconceptions', *Evidence-Based Nursing*, 1,1: 38–9.

Dickie, V. A. 2003. 'Data Analysis in Qualitative Research: A Plea for Sharing the Magic and Effort', *The American Journal of Occupational Therapy*, 57,1: 49–56.

Dixon-Woods, M., Shaw, R. L., Agarwal, S. and Smith, J. A. 2004. 'The Problem of Appraising Qualitative Research', *Quality and Safety in Healthcare*, 13,3: 223–5.

Dixon-Woods, M., Agarwal, S., Jones, D., Young, B. and Sutton, A. 2005. 'Synthesising Qualitative and Quantitative Evidence: A Review of Possible Methods', *Journal of Health Services Research and Policy*, 10,1: 45–53.

Dixon-Woods, M., Bonas, S., Booth, A., Jones, D. R., Miller, T., Sutton, A. J., Shaw, R. L., Smith, J. A. and Young, B. 2006. 'How Can Systematic Reviews Incorporate Qualitative Research? A Critical Perspective', *Qualitative Research*, 6,1:27–44.

Driscoll, D. L., Appiah-Yeboah, A., Salib, B. and Rupert, D. J. 2007. 'Merging Qualitative and Quantitative Data in Mixed Methods Research: How To and Why Not', *Ecological and Environmental Anthropology*, 3,1: 19–28.

Doran, G. T. 1981. 'There's a SMART Way to Write Management's Goals and Objectives', *Management Review*, 70,11: 35–6.

Dowling, M. 2004. 'Hermeneutics: An Exploration', *Nurse Researcher*, 11,4: 30–41.

Duval, S. and Tweedie, R. 2000a. 'A Nonparametric "Trim and Fill" Method of Accounting for Publication Bias in Meta-Analysis', *Journal of the American Statistical Association*, 9,449: 89–98.

Duval, S. and Tweedie, R. 2000b. 'Trim and Fill: A Simple Funnel-Plot-Based Method of Testing and Adjusting for Publication Bias in Meta-Analysis', *Biometrics*, 56, 2: 455–63.

Effken, J. A., Verran, J. A., Logue, M. D. and Hsu, Y. C. 2010. 'Nurse Managers' Decisions: Fast and Favoring Remediation', *Journal of Nursing Administration*, 40,4: 188–95.

Elliot, J. 2005. *Using Narrative in Social Research. Qualitative and Quantitative Approaches*. London: Sage Publications.

Estabrooks, C. A., Field, P. A. and Morse, J. M. 1994. 'Aggregating Qualitative Findings: An Approach to Theory Development', *Qualitative Health Research*, 4,4: 503–11.

Flemming, K. 1998. 'Asking Answerable Questions', *Evidence-Based Nursing*, 1,2: 36–7.

Flemming, K. 2007. 'The Knowledge Base for Evidence-Based Nursing: A Role for Mixed Methods Research?', *Advances in Nursing Science*, 30,1: 41–51.

Fossey, E., Harvey, C., McDermott, F. and Davidson, L. 2002. 'Understanding and Evaluating Qualitative Research', *Australian and New Zealand Journal of Psychiatry*, 36,6: 717–32.

Gallant, M. H., Beaulieu, M. C., Carnevale, F. A. 2002. 'Partnership: An Analysis of the Concept within the Nurse-Client Relationship', *Journal of Advanced Nursing*, 40,2: 149–57.

Gerrish, K. and Clayton, J. 2004. 'Promoting Evidence-Based Practice: An Organizational Approach', *Journal of Nursing Management*, 12,2: 114–23.

Giddings, L. S. and Grant, B. M. 2007. 'A Trojan Horse for Positivism? A Critique of Mixed Methods Research', *Advances in Nursing Science*, 30,1: 52–60.

Gifford, W., Davies, B., Edwards, N., Griffin, P. and Lybanon, V. 2007. 'Managerial Leadership for Nurses' Use of Research Evidence: An Integrative Review of the Literature', *Worldviews Evidence Based Nursing*, 4,3: 126–45.

Glasziou, P., Vandenbroucke, J. and Chalmers, P. 2004. 'Assessing the Quality of Research', *British Medical Journal*, 328,7430: 39–41.

Golden, B. 2006. 'Transforming Healthcare Organizations', *Healthcare Quarterly*, 10, (sp): 10–19.

Goodman, B. 2008. 'Crunch the Numbers', *Nursing Standard*, 22,29: 49.

Graneheim, U. H. and Lundman, B. 2004. 'Qualitative Content Analysis in Nursing Research: Concepts, Procedures and Measures to Achieve Trustworthiness', *Nurse Education Today*, 24,2: 105–12.

Green, S., Higgins, J. T. P., Alderson, P., Clarke, M., Mulrow, C. D. and Oxman, A. D. 2009. 'Introduction', J. T. P. Higgins And S. Green (eds), *Cochrane Handbook for Systematic Reviews of Interventions, Version 5.0.2*. The Cochrane Collaboration. Available from www.cochrane-handbook.org.

Greenhalgh, T. 2010. 'Statistics for the Non-Statistician', in *How to Read a Paper: The Basics of Evidence-Based Medicine*, 4th edn. Chichester: Wiley-Blackwell, pp. 61–76.

Groenwold, R. H. H., Rovers, M. M., Lubsen, J. and Van der Heijden, G. J. M. G. 2010. 'Subgroup Effects Despite Homogeneous Heterogeneity Test Results', *BMC Medical Research Methodology*, 10,43. Available at http://www.biomedcentral.com/1471-2288/10/43; accessed 24 September 2010.

Grol, R. and Grimashaw, J. 2003. 'From Best Evidence to Best Practice: Effective Implementation of Change in a Patients' Care', *The Lancet*, 362,9391: 1225–30.

Guo, K. L. 2008. 'DECIDE: A Decision-Making Model for More Effective Decision Making by Health Care Managers', *The Health Care Manager*, 27,2: 118–27.

Hahn, D. L. 2009. 'Importance of Evidence Grading for Guideline Implementation: The Example of Asthma', *Annals of Family Medicine*, 7,4: 364–9.

Halcomb, E. J., Andrew, S. and Brannen, J. 2009. 'Introduction to Mixed Methods Research for Nursing and the Health Sciences', in S. Andrews and E. J. Halcomb (eds), *Mixed Methods Research for Nursing and the Health Sciences*. Chichester: Wiley-Blackwell Publishing, pp. 3–12.

Hand, H. 2003. 'The Mentor's Tale: A Reflexive Account of Semi Structured Interviews', *Nurse Researcher*, 10,3: 15–27.

Happ, B. H., Dabbs, A. D., Tate, J., Hrick, A. and Erlen, J. 2006. 'Exemplars of Mixed Methods Data Combination and Analysis', *Nursing Research*, 55,2S: S43–9.

Hart, P., Eaton, L. A., Buckner, M., Morrow, B. M., Barrett, D. T., Fraser, D. D., Hooks, D. and Sharer, R. L. 2008. 'Effectiveness of a Computer-Based Educational Program on Nurses' Knowledge, Attitude, and Skill Level Related to Evidence-Based Practice', *Worldviews on Evidence Based Nursing*, 5,2: 75–84.

Haveri, A. 2008. 'Evaluation of Change in Local Governance: The Rhetorical Wall and the Politics of Images', *Evaluation*, 14,2: 141–55.

Hedberg, B. and Larsson, U. S. 2003. 'Observations, Confirmations and Strategies – Useful Tools in Decision-Making Process for Nurses in Practice?', *Journal of Clinical Nursing*, 12,2: 215–22.

Hemingway, P. and Brereton, N. 2009. *What is a Systematic Review?* 2nd edn. Hayward Medical Communications. http://www.whatisseries.co.uk/whatis/pdfs/What_is_syst_rev.pdf; accessed 2 September 2010.

Hebda, T. and Czar, P. 2009. *Handbook of Informatics for Nurses and Healthcare Professionals*. 4th edn. Upper Saddle River, New Jersey, USA: Pearson Education Inc.

Hewitt-Taylor, J. 2006. *Clinical Guidelines and Care Protocols*. Chichester: Wiley.

Hill, T. and Lewicki, P. 2007. *Statistics Methods and Applications*. Tulsa OK, USA: Statsoft.

Holland, M. 2007. *Advanced Searching: Researcher Guide*. Bournemouth: Bournemouth University.

Hoye, S. and Severinsson, E. 2007. 'Methodological Aspects of Rigor in Qualitative Nursing Research on Families Involved in Intensive Care Units: A Literature Review', *Nursing and Health Sciences*, 9,1: 61–8.

Hu, W., Kemp, A. and Kerridge, I. 2004. 'Making Clinical Decisions When the Stakes are High and the Evidence Unclear', *British Medical Journal*, 329,7470: 852–4.

Hughes, R. 2008. 'Understanding Audit: Methods and Application', *Nursing and Residential Care*, 11,2 :88–91.

Hutchinson, A. M. and Johnston, I. 2004. 'Bridging the Divide: A Survey of Nurses' Opinions Regarding Barriers to, and Facilitators of, Research Utilization in the Practice Setting', *Journal of Clinical Nursing*, 13,3: 304–15.

Jadad, A. R. 2002. 'Evidence-Based Decision Making and Asthma in the Internet Age: The Tools of the Trade', *Allergy*, 57,74: 15–22.

Jamieson, S. 2004. 'Likert Scales, How to (Ab)Use Them', *Medical Education*, 38,12: 1217–18.

Johnson, R. B. and Onwuegbuzie, A. J. 2004. 'Mixed Methods Research: A Research Paradigm whose Time Has Come', *Educational Researcher*, 33,7: 14–26.

Jootun, D. and McGhee, G. 2009. 'Reflexivity: Promoting Rigour in Qualitative Research', *Nursing Standard*, 23,2: 42–6.

Kaplan, C. 2002. 'Children and the Law: The Place of Health Professionals', *Child and Adolescent Mental Health*, 7,4: 181–8.

Karlsson, U. and Tornquist, K. 2007. 'What Do Swedish Occupational Therapists Feel about Research? A Survey of Perceptions, Attitudes, Intentions, and Engagement', *Scandinavian Journal of Occupational Therapy*, 14,4: 221–9.

Kearney, M. H. 2005. 'Seeking the Sound Bite: Reading and Writing Clinically Useful Qualitative Research', *Journal of Obstetric, Gynecologic and Neonatal Nursing*, 34,4: 417.

Kegan, R. and Lahey, L. L. 2001. 'The Real Reason People Won't Change', *Harvard Business Review*, November: 85–92.

Kennedy, I. 2003. 'Patients are Experts in their Own Field', *British Medical Journal*, 326,7402: 1276–7.

King, G., Currie, M., Bartlett, D. J., Strachan, D., Tucker, M. A. and Willoughby, C. 2008. 'The Development of Expertise in Paediatric Rehabilitation Therapists: The Roles of Motivation, Openness to Experience, and Types of Caseload Experience', *Australian Occupational Therapy Journal*, 55,2: 108–22.

King, L. and Clark, J. M. 2002. 'Intuition and the Development of Expertise in Surgical Ward and Intensive Care Nurses', *Journal of Advanced Nursing*, 37,4: 322–9.

Koch, T. 2006. 'Establishing Rigour in Qualitative Research: The Decision Trail', *Journal of Advanced Nursing*, 53,1: 91–100.

Kuuppelomaki, M. and Tuomi, J. 2005. 'Finnish Nurses' Attitudes towards Nursing Research and Related Factors', *International Journal of Nursing Studies*, 42,2: 187–96.

Le May, 2001. *Making Use of Research*. London: Distance Learning Centre, South Bank University.

Lee, P. 2006a. 'Understanding and Critiquing Quantitative Research Papers', *Nursing Times*, 102,28:28–30.

Lee, P. 2006b. 'Understanding and Critiquing Qualitative Research Papers' *Nursing Times*, 102,29:30–2.

Lee, P. 2006c. 'Understanding the Basic Aspects of Research Papers', *Nursing Times*, 102,27: 28–30.

Lefebvre, C., Manheimer, E. and Glanville, J. 2009. 'Searching for Studies', in J. T. P. Higgins and S. Green (eds), *Cochrane Handbook for Systematic Reviews of Interventions. Version 5.0.2*. The Cochrane Collaboration. www.cochrane-handbook.org.

Lemmer, B., Steven, J. and Grellier, R. 1998. 'Decision-Making: A Study of Influences on Health Visitors', *Community Practitioner*, 71,11: 368–70.

Lewin, K. 1951. *Field Theory in Social Science Selected Theoretical Papers*. New York, Harper and Row.

Lincoln, Y. S. and Guba, E. G. 1985. *Naturalistic Inquiry*. Newbury Park, California: Sage Publications.

Liu, J., Wyatt, J. C. and Altman, D. G. 2006. 'Decision Tools in Health Care: Focus on the Problem, Not the Solution', *BMC Medical Informatics and Decision Making*, 6,4, available at http://www.biomedcentral.com/1472-6947/6/4; accessed 4 September 2010.

Lo Bindo-Wood, G. and Haber, J. 2005. *Nursing Research Methods and Critical Appraisal for Evidence Based Practice. 6th edn*. St Louis Missouri, USA: Mosby Elsevier.

Lopez, K. and Willis, D. 2004. 'Descriptive versus Interpretive Phenomenology: Their Contributions to Nursing Knowledge', *Qualitative Health Research*, 14,5: 726–35.

Lowden, J. 2002. 'Children's Rights: A Decade of Dispute', *Journal of Advanced Nursing*, 37,1: 100–7.

Ludwick, D. A. and Doucette, J. 2009. 'The Implementation of Operational Processes for the Alberta Electronic Health Record: Lessons from Electrical Medical Record Adoption in Primary Care', *Healthcare Quarterly*, 12,2: 103–7.

Lyneham, J., Parkinson, C. and Denholm, C. 2009. 'Expert Nursing Practice: A Mathematical Explanation of Benner's 5th Stage of Practice Development', *Journal of Advanced Nursing*, 65,11: 2477–84.

McAuley, C., McCurry, N., Knapp, M., Beecham, J., and Sleed, M. 2006. 'Young Families under Stress: Assessing Maternal and Child Well-Being Using a Mixed-Methods Approach', *Child and Family Social Work*, 11,1: 43–54.

McBrien, B. 2008. 'Evidence-Based Care: Enhancing the Rigour of Qualitative Study', *British Journal of Nursing*, 17,20: 1286–9.

McGrath, J. E. and Johnson, B. A. 2003. 'Methodology Makes Meaning: How Both Qualitative and Quantitative Paradigms Shape Evidence and its Interpretation', in P. M. Camic, J. E. Rhodes and L. Yardley (eds), *Qualitative Research in Psychology: Expanding Perspectives in Methodology and Design*. Washington DC: APA Books, pp. 31–8.

MacInnes, J. 2009. 'Mixed Methods Studies: A Guide to Critical Appraisal', *British Journal of Cardiac Nursing*, 4,12: 588–91.

Maltby, J., Williams, G.A., McGarry, J. and Day, L. 2010. *Research Methods for Nursing and Healthcare*. Harlow: Pearson Education.

Martin, C. 2002. 'The Theory of Critical Thinking of Nursing', *Nursing Education Perspectives*, 23,5: 243–7.

Mertens, D. M. 2005. *Research and Evaluation in Education and Psychology: Integrating Diversity with Quantitative, Qualitative and Mixed Methods*, 2nd edn. Thousand Oaks California, USA: Sage Publications.

Moran, J. W. and Brightman, B. K. 1998. 'Effective Management of Healthcare Change', *The TQM Magazine*, 10,1: 27–9.

Moreno, S. G., Sutton, A. J., Turner, E. H., Abrams, K. R., Cooper, N. J., Palmer, T. M. and Ades, A. E. 2009. 'Novel Methods to Deal with Publication Biases: Secondary Analysis of Antidepressant Trials in the FDA Trial Registry Database and Related Journal Publications', *British Medical Journal*, 339,7719: 493–8.

Morgan, D. 2007. 'Paradigms Lost and Pragmatism Regained: Methodological Implications of Combing Qualitative and Quantitative Methods', *Journal of Mixed Methods Research*, 1,1: 48–76.

Morris-Docker, S. B., Tod A. Harrison, J. H., Wolstenholme, D. and Black, R. 2004. 'Nurses' Use of the Internet in Clinical Ward Settings', *Journal of Advanced Nursing*, 48,2: 157–66.

Morse, J. M. 2003. 'Principles of Mixed Methods and Multimethod Research Design', in A. Tashakkori and C. B. Teddlie (eds), *Handbook of Mixed Methods in Social and Behavioral Research*. Thousand Oaks, California, USA: Sage Publications, pp. 189–208.

Motulsky, H. 1995. *Intuitive Biostatistics*. Oxford: Oxford University Press.

Murphy, S. L., Robinson, J. C. and Lin, S. H. 2009. 'Conducting Systematic Reviews to Inform Occupational Therapy Practice', *The American Journal of Occupational Therapy*, 68,3: 363–8.

Mylopoulos, M. and Regehr, G. 2009. 'How Student Models of Expertise and Innovation Impact the Development of Adaptive Expertise in Medicine', *Medical Education*, 43,2: 127–32.

National Institute for Health and Clinical Excellence. 2005. *Assessing Evidence and Recommendations in NICE Guidelines – Paper for SMT*. www. nice.org.uk/niceMedia/pdf/smt/?251005item3.pdf; accessed 9 September 2010.

National Patient Safety Agency and Research Ethics Service. 2008. *Defining Research. Issue 3*. London: National Patient Safety Agency.

Nelson, A. M. 2002. A Metasynthesis: Mothering Other-Than-Normal Children', *Qualitative Health Research*, 12,4: 515–30.

Nojima, Y., Tomikawa Makabe, S. and Snyder, M. 2003. 'Defining Characteristics of Expertise in Japanese Clinical Nursing Using the Delphi Technique', *Nursing and Health Sciences*, 5,1: 3–11.

Onwuegbuzie, A. J. and Johnson, R. B. 2006. 'The Validity Issue in Mixed Research', *Research in the Schools*, 13,1: 48–63.

Orfali, K. and Gordon, E. 2004. 'Autonomy Gone Awry: A Cross-Cultural Study of Parents' Experiences in Neonatal Intensive Care Units', *Theoretical Medicine and Bioethics*, 25,4: 329–65.

Oxman, A. D. and Flottorp, S. 2001. 'An Overview of Strategies to Promote Implementation of Evidence-Based Health Care', in C. Silagy and A. Haines (eds), *Evidence-Based Practice in Primary Care*. 2nd edn. London: BMJ books, pp. 101–19.

Parahoo, K. 2006. *Nursing Research: Principles, Process and Issues*. 2nd edn. Basingstoke: Palgrave Macmillan.

Paul, W. P. and Heaslip, P. 1995. 'Critical Thinking and Intuitive Nursing Practice', *Journal of Advanced Nursing*, 22,1: 40–7.

Pearcey, P. and Draper, P. 1996. 'Using the Diffusion of Innovation Model to Influence Practice: A Case Study', *Journal of Advanced Nursing*, 23,4: 714–21.

Piderit, S. K. 2000. 'Rethinking Resistance and Recognizing Ambivalence: A Multidimensional View of Attitudes Toward an Organizational Change', *Academy of Management Review*, 25, 4: 783–94.

Polit, D. F. and Beck, C. T. 2006. *Essentials of Nursing Research: Methods, Appraisal and Utilisation*. 6th edn. Philadelphia PA USA: Lippincott Williams and Wilkins.

Polkinghorne, D. E. 2005. 'Language and Meaning: Data Collection in Qualitative Research', *Journal of Counselling Psychology*, 52,2: 137–45.

Ponterotto, J. G. 2005.'Qualitative Research in Counselling Psychology: A Primer on Research Paradigms and Philosophy of Science', *Journal of Counselling Psychology*, 52,2: 126–36.

Price, B. 2008. 'Strategies to Help Nurses Cope with Change in the Healthcare Setting', *Nursing Standard*, 22,48: 50–6.

Prochaska, J. O. and DiClemente, C. C. 1992. 'Stages of Change in the Modification of Problem Behaviours', *Progress in Behaviour Modification*, 28: 183–218.

Protheroe, J. Fahey. T., Montgomery, A. A. and Peters, T. J. 2000. 'The Impact of Patients' Preferences on the Treatment of Atrial Fibrillation: Observational

Study of Patient-Based Decision Analysis', *British Medical Journal*, 320,7246: 1380–4.

Pryjmachuk, S. 1996. 'Pragmatism and Change: Some Implications for Nurses, Nurse Managers and Nursing', *Journal of Nursing Management*, 4,4: 201–5.

Rassafian, M. 2009. 'Is Length of Experience an Appropriate Criterion to Identify Level of Expertise?', *Scandinavian Journal of Occupational Therapy*, 16,4: 247–56.

Reed, J. and Turner, J. 2005. 'Appreciating Change in Cancer services – An Evaluation of Service Development Strategies', *Journal of Health Organization and Management*, 19,2: 163–76.

Reid, G., Kneafsey, R., Long, A., Hulme, C. and Wright, H. 2007. 'Change and Transformation: The Impact of an Action-Research Evaluation on the Development of a New Service', *Learning in Health and Social Care*, 6,2: 61–71.

Ren, D. 2009. 'Understanding Statistical Hypothesis Testing', *Journal of Emergency Nursing*, 35,1: 57–9.

Richens, Y., Rycroft-Malone, J. and Morrell, C. 2004. 'Getting Guidelines into Practice: A Literature Review', *Nursing Standard*, 18,50: 33–40.

Roberts, P. and Priest, H. 2006. 'Reliability and Validity in Research', *Nursing Standard*, 20,44: 41–5.

Rodgers, M., Sowden, A., Petticrew, M., Arai, L., Roberts, H., Britten, N. and Popay, J. 2009. 'Testing Methodological Guidance on the Conduct of Narrative Synthesis in Systematic Reviews', *Evaluation*, 15,1: 47–71.

Rogers, E. M. 1995. *Diffusion of Innovations*, 4th edn. New York: Free Press.

Rolfe, G., Segrott, J. and Jordan, S. 2008. 'Tensions and Contradictions in Nurses' Perspectives of Evidence-Based Practice', *Journal of Nursing Management*, 16,4: 440–51.

Russell, C. L. 2005. 'Evaluating Quantitative Research Reports', *Nephrology Nursing*, 32,1:61–4.

Russell, C. K. and Gregory, D. M. 2003. 'Evaluation of Qualitative Research Studies', *Evidence-Based Nursing*, 6,2:36–40.

Ryan, F., Coughlan, M. and Cronin, P. 2007 'Step-byStep Guide to Critiquing Research. Part 2: Qualitative Research', *British Journal of Nursing*, 16,12: 738–44.

Sackett, D. L., Rosenberg, W. M. C., Gray, J. A. M., Haynes, R. B. and Richardson, W. S. 1996. 'Evidence-Based Medicine: What it is and What it isn't', *British Medical Journal*, 312,7023:71–2.

Saba, V. K. and McCormick, K. A. 2001. *Essentials of Computers for Nurses*. 3rd edn. New York, USA: McGraw-Hill.

Sale, J. E. M., Lohnfeld, L. H. and Brazil, K. 2002. 'Revisiting the Quantitative-Qualitative Debate: Implications for Mixed Methods Research', *Quality and Quantity* 36,1: 43–5.

Sale, J. E. M. and Brazil, K. 2004. 'A Strategy to Identify Critical Appraisal Criteria for Primary Mixed-Method Studies', *Quality and Quantity*, 38,4: 351–65.

Sandelowski, M. 2004. 'Using Qualitative Research', *Qualitative Health Research*, 14,10: 1366–86.

Sandelowski, M. and Barroso, J. 2002. 'Finding the Findings in Qualitative Studies', *Journal of Nursing*, 34,3: 213–19.

Saull-McCaig, S., Pacheco, R., Kozak, P., Gauthier, S. and Hahn, R. 2006. 'Implementing MOE/MAR: Balancing Project Management with Change Management', *Healthcare Quarterly*, 10(Sp): 27–38.

Schreiber, R. Crooks, D. and Stern, P. N. 1997. 'Qualitative Meta-Analysis', in J. M. Morse (ed.), *Completing a Qualitative Project: Details and Dialogue*. Thousand Oaks, California, USA: Sage, pp. 311–26.

Scott, T., Mannion, R., Marshall, M. and Davies, H. 2003. 'Does Organizational Culture Influence Healthcare Performance? A Review of the Evidence', *Journal of Health Services Research and Policy*, 8,2: 105–17.

Scott, S., Estabrooks, C. and Allen M. Pollock, C. 2008. 'A Context of Uncertainty: How Context Shapes Nurses' Research Utilisation Behaviours', *Qualitative Health Research*, 18,3: 347–57.

Scottish Intercollegiate Guidelines Network (SIGN). 2010.*Management of Obesity: A National Clinical Guideline*. Edinburgh: SIGN.

Sitzia, J. 2002. 'Barriers to Research Utilisation: The Clinical Setting and Nurses Themselves', *Intensive and Critical Care Nursing*, 18,4: 230–43.

Skinner, D. 2004. 'Evaluation and Change Management: Rhetoric and Reality', *Human Resources Management Journal*, 14,3: 5–19.

SOA.com. 2001. *Search Engine* http://searchsoa.techtarget.com/sDefinition/0,,sid26_gci212955,00.html; accessed 24 September 2010.

Standing, M. 2007. 'Clinical Decision-Making Skills on the Developmental Journey from Student to Registered Nurse: A longitudinal Inquiry', *Journal of Advanced Nursing*, 60,3: 257–69.

Stanley, D. 2004. 'Clinical Leaders in Paediatric Nursing: A Pilot Study', *Paediatric Nursing*, 16,3: 39–42.

Stoller, J. K., Sasidhar, M., Wheeler, D.M., Chatburn, R. L., Bivens, R. T., Priganc, D. and Orens, D. K. 2010. 'Team-Building and Change Management in Respiratory Care: Description of a Process and Outcomes', *Respiratory Care*, 55,6:741–8.

Tarling, M. and Crofts, L. 2000. *The Essential Researcher's Handbook*. London: Balliere Tindall.

Tashakkori, A. and Creswell, J. W. 2007. 'The New Era of Mixed Methods', *Journal of Mixed Methods Research*, 1,1: 3–7.

Tashakkori, A. and Teddlie, C. 2003. *Handbook of Mixed Methods in Social and Behavioral Research*. Thousand Oaks, California, USA: Sage Publications.

Teddlie, C. and Yu, F. 2007. 'Mixed Methods Sampling: A Typology with Examples', *Journal of Mixed Methods Research*, 1,1: 77–100.

Thames Valley Literature Review Standards Group. 2006. *The Literature Searching Process: Protocol for Researchers*. London: Thames Valley Health Libraries Network.

Thomas, E. 2004. 'An Introduction to Medical Statistics for Health Care Professionals: Describing and Presenting Data', *Musculoskeletal Care*, 4,2: 218–28.

Thomas, E. 2005. 'An Introduction to Medical Statistics for Health Care Professionals: Hypothesis Tests and Estimation', *Musculoskeletal Care*, 3,2: 102–8.

Thompson, C., McCaughan, D., Cullum, N., Sheldon, T., Thompson, D. and Mulhall, A. 2001. *Nurses' Use of Research Information in Clinical Decision Making: A Descriptive and Analytical Study. Final Report. NHS R & D Programme in Evaluating Methods to Promote the Implementation of R & D.* London: Department of Health.

Thompson, D. R., Chau, J. P. C., Lopez, V. 2006. 'Barriers to, and Facilitators of, Research Utilisation: A Survey of Hong Kong Registered Nurses', *International Journal of Evidence-Based Healthcare*, 4, 2: 77–82.

Thorne, S. and Darbyshire, P. 2005. 'Land Mines in the Field: A Modest Proposal for Improving the Craft of Qualitative Health Research', *Qualitative Health Research*, 15,8: 1105–13.

Thorne, S., Paterson, B., Acorn, S., Canam, C., Joachim, G. and Jillings, C. 2002. 'Chronic Illness Experience: Insights from a Metastudy', *Qualitative Health Research*, 12,4: 437–52.

Tobin, G. A. and Begley, C. M. 2004. 'Methodological Rigour within a Qualitative Framework', *Journal of Advanced Nursing*, 48,4: 388–96.

Todres, L. 2005. 'Clarifying the Life-World: Descriptive Phenomenology', in I. Holloway (ed.), *Qualitative Research in Healthcare*. Maidenhead: Open University Press, pp. 104–24.

Van Bokhoven, M. A., Kok, G. and van der Weijden, T. 2003. 'Designing a Quality Improvement Intervention: A Systematic Approach', *Quality and Safety in Healthcare*, 12,3: 215–20.

Vevea, J. L. and Woods, C. M. 2005. 'Publication Bias in Research Synthesis: Sensitivity Analysis Using a Priori Weight Functions', *Psychological Methods*, 10,4: 428–43.

Vishnevsky, T. and Beanlands, H. 2004. 'Qualitative Research', *Nephrology Nursing Journal*, 31,2: 234–8.

Wade, D. T. 2005. 'Ethics, Audit and Research: All Shades of Grey', *British Medical Journal*, 330,7489: 468–71.

Webber, J. 2009. 'Building Professional Nursing', in W. L. Holzemer (ed.), *Improving Health through Nursing Research*. Chichester: Wiley-Blackwell, pp. 52–66.

Whiting, L.S. 2008. 'Semi-Structured Interviews: Guidance for Novice Researchers', *Nursing Standard*, 22,23: 35–40.

Willig, C. 2008. *Introducing Qualitative Research in Psychology. Adventures in Theory and Method.* 2nd edn. Maidenhead: Open University Press.

Wilmot, S. 2003. *Ethics, Power and Policy: The Future of Nursing in the NHS.* Basingstoke: Palgrave Macmillan.

Windish, D. M. and Diener-West, M. 2006. 'A Clinician-Educator's Roadmap to Choosing and Interpreting Statistical Tests', *Journal of General Internal Medicine*, 21,6: 656–60.

Wood, M. J., Ross-Kerr, J. C. and Brink, P. J. 2006. *Basic Steps in Planning Nursing Research: From Question to Proposal*, 6th edn. Sudbury: Jones and Bartlett.

Wright, S. 2010. 'Dealing with Resistance', *Nursing Standard*, 24,23: 18–20.

Zimmer, L. 2006. 'Qualitative Meta-Synthesis: A Question of Dialoguing with Texts', *Journal of Advanced Nursing*, 53,3: 311–18.

Zondervan, K. T. Cardon, L. R. and Kennedy, S. H. 2002. 'What Makes a Good Case-Control Study? Design Issues for Complex Traits Such as Endometriosis', *Human Reproduction*, 7,6: 1415–23.

Index

Action plan 130–131, 134, 149, 163
Aggregative synthesis 105
Alternate hypothesis 47
Anonymity 37, 42, 76, 86, 87, 92, 93, 160
ANOVA 56, 57, 162
Applicability of studies 7, 14, 30, 40, 59, 60, 76, 79, 107, 108, 109, 120, 121
Appraising research: principles 29–45
Appraising research: qualitative 65–80
Appraising research: quantitative 46–64
Approaches to evaluating change 148–151
Audit 11–12, 38
Auditability 75, 78, 106
Autonomy 36, 37, 119, 120, 154, 155
Axiology 13

Barriers to change 128, 134, 135–138
Bell curve 53, 54
Beneficence 36
Benefits of using research 3–5
Bias 31, 33, 44, 49, 62, 92, 95, 98, 100, 101, 102, 112, 152, 159
Blinding 49, 62
Boolean terms 24–25, 28, 111
Bottom-up change 139

Case control studies 50, 51, 64, 110
Case reports 94, 108, 109, 110
CASP tools 40, 98, 165
Categories 38, 72, 76, 79, 80, 104, 105, 106, 154, 160
Central tendency 55, 63
Challenges of using research 5–7
Changing practice 123–131, 132–145
Changing practice, aims 123–126, 133, 146, 148, 163
Changing practice, objectives 125–126, 133, 148, 152, 163
Changing personal practice 123–131
Changing team practice 132–145
Chi square 56, 57, 62, 63, 64, 93, 162
Clinical evaluation 11–12, 38
Clinical guidelines 95, 107–108, 109, 110, 116
Clinical judgement 116, 117, 121
Cochrane collaboration 21, 165
Codes 38, 72, 73, 75, 79, 88, 93, 106, 154, 160
Coding 37, 38, 72, 73, 75, 79, 88, 93, 106, 154, 160

Conclusions 3, 10, 32, 38, 39, 40, 41, 42, 43, 44, 45, 59, 60, 62, 63, 64, 66, 73, 75, 76, 78, 79, 80, 85, 89, 90, 92, 93, 99, 104, 106, 161
Concurrent mixed methods design 84
Confidence interval 59, 100, 101, 160
Confidence level 101
Confidence limits 59, 100, 101, 160
Confidentiality 37, 43, 79, 80, 87, 93, 155, 160
Confirmability 74, 75
Confounding variables 33, 60, 62
Consent 12, 36, 37, 41, 43, 62, 77, 78, 86, 87, 93, 155, 160
Construct validity 53, 160
Content validity 53, 160
Context of studies 3, 7, 14, 15, 32, 42, 45, 68, 70, 71, 74, 75, 76, 77, 78, 79, 107, 160
Control group 12, 48, 49, 56, 62, 100
Convenience sample 35, 45, 79, 80
Correlation 57
Credibility 74, 75, 78, 161
Criterion validity 53, 160
Cross sectional studies 50, 64

Data analysis 32, 34, 38, 41, 43, 44, 45, 53–59, 61, 62, 63, 64, 72–76, 77, 78, 79, 80, 81, 87–88, 89, 90, 91, 92, 93, 107, 153, 154, 160, 161
Data analysis, mixed methods 87–88, 89, 90, 91, 92, 93, 107, 161
Data analysis, qualitative 38, 41, 43, 72–76, 77, 78, 79, 80, 81, 160, 161
Data analysis, quantitative 45, 53–59, 61, 62, 63, 64, 160
Data bases 19–21, 22, 23, 24, 25, 26, 27, 96, 110, 111, 165
Data saturation 34, 71, 77, 78
Data transformation 72, 88, 90
Decision making 4, 6, 7, 8, 10, 22, 56, 66, 69, 70, 71, 75, 82, 83, 95, 97, 102, 104, 105, 107, 115–122, 138, 140, 141, 143, 144, 145, 162
Deductive coding 72
Defending change 130, 137
Defending decisions 122
Definition of research 9–11
Dependability 74, 75, 78, 161

Decision making tools   121
Descriptive studies   50
Descriptive statistics   45, 54–55, 59, 62, 91, 153, 162
Dissemination   158
Document analysis   67, 70, 149
Driving forces, change   134–135, 140

Eligibility criteria, systematic review   95, 97, 105, 111
Empirical - rational   133, 140
Ethics, research   1, 12, 36–38, 41, 43, 44, 62, 63, 77, 78, 79, 80, 86, 91, 93, 119, 160
Ethics: evaluation   154
Ethnography   15, 67, 70, 84,
Epistemology   13
Evaluation aims   11–12, 129, 146, and 147
Evaluation approaches   148–149
Evaluation of change   7, 129, 146–156
Evaluation data   152
Evaluation methods   149–152
Evaluation, timing   137, 147–148, 153
Evidence based practice   115, 121
Exclusion criteria   34, 53, 61, 97, 98, 99, 102, 103, 105, 106, 111
Experience   115, 116, 117, 118, 120, 121, 122
Experimental studies   47–50, 62
Expert decision making   115–118, 122
Expertise   115–118
Expert opinion   27, 44, 94, 108, 109, 111, 112
External validity   52, 53, 160

Field diary   70
Findings   42, 43, 45, 76, 77, 88–89, 91, 93, 98
Findings, mixed methods   88–89, 91, 93
Findings qualitative   42, 43, 76
Findings quantitative   59–60, 63, 64
Focus group   79, 80, 91, 92
Force field analysis   134–135
Forest plot   100, 101, 103
Frameworks for evaluating research   40, 89, 98, 159, 165

Generalizability   13, 14, 15, 30, 32, 34, 35, 43, 45, 50, 51, 53, 56, 57, 58, 59, 61, 62, 63, 65, 66, 71, 75, 76, 78, 79, 80, 89, 93, 105, 109, 154
Grey literature   96, 101, 111, 158
Group interview   75, 79, 91, 149
Grounded theory   66, 67, 68, 71, 73, 77, 78, 83

Heterogeneity   102–104
Hierarchies of evidence   109–110
Hypothesis   31, 32, 47–48, 56, 57, 58, 61, 62, 63, 64, 66, 83, 159, 161

Inclusion criteria   34, 53, 61, 64, 97, 98, 99, 102, 103, 105, 106, 111

Index of Theses   21
Inductive coding   72, 79
Inferential statistics   54, 56–57, 59, 63, 93, 154, 160, 162
Integrative synthesis   105
Internal validity   52, 160
Interpreting evaluation data   153–154
Interpretivist   13
Interval data   54
Interviews   16, 33, 34, 36, 37, 41, 51, 52, 68, 69, 70, 71, 74, 75, 76, 77, 78, 79, 80, 82, 84, 85, 86, 87, 88, 91, 92, 149
Interviews, face to face   37, 69
Interviews, semi-structured   69
Interviews, structured   69
Interviews, telephone   69
Interviews, unstructured   69

Justice   4, 36, 154

Key players (change)   138–140, 145
Key words   22, 28, 111
Kruskal-Wallis test   57, 162

Literature review   31–32, 53, 66–67, 83–84, 159
Longitudinal studies   50

Maintaining change   142
Management involvement in change   139, 142–143
Mann-Whitney test   57, 64, 162
Mean   44, 45, 54, 55, 56, 57, 59, 162
Median   55, 57, 64, 162
Member checking   74–75, 78, 80, 92
Meta analysis   98, 99–104, 107, 108, 109, 110, 111, 112
Meta synthesis   98, 99, 104–107, 108, 110, 111
Methodology   13, 15, 16, 32, 33, 34, 40, 41, 44, 48–51, 61, 62, 63, 64, 66, 67–68, 72, 77, 78, 79, 80, 82, 83, 84–85, 89, 90, 91, 92, 95, 106, 107, 159, 161
Methodology, qualitative   15, 16, 32, 33, 41, 42, 67–68, 72, 77, 78, 79, 80
Methodology, quantitative   16, 32, 44, 48–51, 61, 62, 63, 64, 66
Methodology, mixed methods   82, 83, 84–85, 89, 90, 91, 92
Methods of evaluation   149–152
Methods of research   15–16, 31, 32–33, 38, 41, 42, 43, 44, 51–52, 61, 63, 68–72, 74, 77, 78, 79, 80, 85–86, 90, 91, 92, 93, 97, 159, 161
Missing data   45, 60, 102, 160
Missing results   60, 160
Mixed methods research   10, 14, 31, 41, 81–93, 107, 161
Mixed method synthesis   107, 108

Mode 55, 162
Motivation 7, 124, 127, 128, 133, 138, 139, 142
Multidisciplinary change management 143–145

Narrative research 67, 68
Narrative synthesis 99, 107, 111
Naturalistic research 13
NICE 21, 27, 108, 110, 111
Nominal data 45, 53, 54, 55, 64
Non-maleficence 36
Non-parametric data 53, 54, 56, 57, 62, 63, 64, 93, 160, 162
Non-parametric tests 53, 54, 56, 57, 62, 63, 64, 93, 160, 162
Non-probability sampling 35–36
Normal distribution curve 53, 54
Normative re-educative 133
Null hypothesis 47, 48, 57, 58, 61, 62, 64

Observation 16, 33, 51 67, 68, 69, 70, 84, 87, 88, 116, 149
Observation: participant 67, 69, 70
Observation: non-participant 69
Observational research 48, 49–51
Observational studies 49–51
Odds ratio 100, 101
One tailed test 57
Ontology 13
Ordinal data 45, 53, 54, 55

P value 57–58, 59, 60, 76, 160
Paradigm 13–15, 16, 32, 34, 40, 44, 78, 82, 83, 88, 90, 104, 159
Paradigm, mixed methods 14, 82, 88, 90
Paradigm, qualitative 13, 14, 15, 16, 32, 78, 82
Paradigm, quantitative 13, 15, 32, 34, 44, 82
Paradigm, pragmatic: see paradigm mixed methods
Parametric data 53, 54, 55, 160, 162
Parametric tests 53, 54, 55, 56, 57, 160, 162
Patient experience 116, 118–120
Patient expertise 116, 120
Patient opinion 116, 120, 121, 122
Patient preferences 116, 118–120, 121, 122
Percentage values 55, 59, 63, 63, 88, 91, 92, 153, 162
Phenomenology 15, 16, 42, 67, 70
Planning change 123, 125, 126, 127, 128, 129, 130, 131, 132, 134, 137, 142, 144, 149, 150, 155, 157
PICO 95, 96, 111
Positivist 13
Power calculation 51, 57, 58, 62, 64
Power-coercive 133, 134
Probability sampling 34–35, 51
Prospective studies 50, 63, 64

Publication bias 101–102
Published research 21, 29, 30, 75, 96
Purposive sampling 35, 71, 80

Qualitative research 13–14, 15, 16, 31, 32, 33, 34, 35, 38, 39, 40, 41, 42, 43, 51, 52, 65–80, 104, 105, 106, 109, 110, 111, 160, 161
Quality, mixed methods 89–90
Quantitative research 13, 14, 15, 31, 32, 33, 34, 35, 38, 40, 41, 44, 46–64, 65, 73, 75, 76, 98, 99, 101, 104, 105, 109, 111, 160
Quasi experimental studies 50
Questionnaires 33, 34, 36, 43, 44, 45, 51, 52, 53, 68, 70, 83, 84, 85, 86, 87, 88, 91, 92, 93, 149

Random sampling 12, 34–35, 51, 52
Randomization 12, 35, 48, 49, 61, 62, 64
Randomized controlled trial (RCT) 10, 49, 61, 95, 96, 98, 99
Ratio data 54, 55
Readiness for change 140–141, 142, 143, 144, 145
Recommendations 3,6, 12, 30, 32, 38, 39, 40, 43, 44, 45, 58, 60, 70, 73, 79, 80, 89, 92, 93, 98, 99, 100, 101, 104, 107, 109, 112, 161
Reflection 70, 117, 118, 122
Reflexivity 118
Regression 57, 102, 103, 104
Reliability 38–39, 52, 64, 92, 160
Research journal 70
Research problem 3 1, 47, 159
Research purpose 36, 47, 51, 53, 61, 63, 66, 83, 89, 159, 161
Research question 31, 32, 47, 64, 66, 72, 76, 83, 85, 159, 161
Research statement 31, 47, 83, 159, 161
Resistance to change 135, 136, 137, 138, 139, 141, 150
Resources 4, 20, 97, 111, 120, 127, 127, 137, 142, 143, 152, 154, 155, 158, 163
Respondent validation 74–75, 78, 80, 92
Response rate 36, 43, 45, 91, 92, 93, 159
Restraining forces (change) 134, 135, 138
Results 10, 32, 34, 35, 36, 37, 38, 39, 40, 41, 44, 45, 47, 48, 49, 50, 52, 56, 57, 59, 60, 62, 64, 75, 80, 92, 97, 100, 101, 103, 104, 111, 152, 156, 159, 160, 161
Retrospective 50, 63, 64
Risk ratio 100

Sampling 33–36, 45, 51, 52, 55, 71–72, 74, 80, 82, 86, 88, 92, 161
Sampling mixed methods 82, 86, 88, 92
Sampling qualitative 34, 35, 71–72, 74, 80
Sampling quantitative 34–35, 51, 52, 55
Search engine 20, 21, 22, 110, 111
Search strategy 96–97

Search terms   23, 27, 28
Search fields   26, 28
Searching for information   5, 16, 19–28
Sensitivity analysis   104
Sequence of evaluation   146–147
Sequential mixed methods design   84, 87, 91
Simultaneous mixed methods design: see concurrent mixed methods design
Snowball sampling   35, 71
Standard deviation   55, 162
Statistical tests   38, 46, 47, 51, 53, 56–59, 61, 87, 88, 100, 102, 103, 160, 162
Subjectivity   10, 14, 32, 65, 73, 74, 99, 109
Summaries of evidence   94–113
Sustaining change   131, 141, 142, 145, 153
Systematic review   95–107, 108

Tails (tests)   57
T test   56, 57, 162
Thematic analysis   43, 77, 87, 91, 93, 104
Themes   42, 43, 72, 76, 77, 78, 79, 80, 88, 91, 98, 105, 106, 154, 160

Timetable for change   129
Top-Down change   139
Tools for evaluating research   40, 89, 98, 159, 165
Transferability   63, 74, 75, 77, 78, 89, 160, 161
Triangulation   70, 74, 85, 106
Truncation   25, 2, 28
Trustworthiness   39, 74, 78, 160, 161
Two tailed test   57
Type I error   57– 58
Type II error   57, 58

Validity   36, 38–9, 44, 52–53, 64, 92, 95, 160
Value of research   3–5
Variables   33, 47, 56, 57, 60, 62, 64, 82, 148, 162
Volunteer sample   35, 36, 37, 42, 43, 79, 80, 92, 151,

Weighting in mixed methods   85
Wilcoxon's test   57, 64, 93,162
Wildcards   25, 26

CPSIA information can be obtained
at www.ICGtesting.com
Printed in the USA
LVOW10s2114271216

518859LV00006B/92/P